VIROLOGY RESEARCH PROGRESS

HEMORRHAGIC FEVER

EPIDEMIOLOGY, CLINICAL MANIFESTATIONS AND DIAGNOSIS

VIROLOGY RESEARCH PROGRESS

Additional books in this series can be found on Nova's website under the Series tab.

Additional e-books in this series can be found on Nova's website under the e-book tab.

VIROLOGY RESEARCH PROGRESS

HEMORRHAGIC FEVER

EPIDEMIOLOGY, CLINICAL MANIFESTATIONS AND DIAGNOSIS

SHIRLEY R. EDWARDS
EDITOR

NOVA BIOMEDICAL
New York

NOTICE TO THE READER

Library of Congress Cataloging-in-Publication Data

ISBN: 978-1-63482-791-1
Library of Congress Control Number: 2015938203

Published by Nova Science Publishers, Inc. † New York

Contents

Preface

Viral hemorrhagic fevers (VHFs) represent a collection of illnesses caused by several distinct viral families. While some types of hemorrhagic fever viruses can cause relatively mild illnesses, many of these viruses cause life-threatening diseases. The chapters of this book discuss the consequences of the Ebola outbreak in West Africa; the most frequency imported infection worldwide (malaria); the reservoirs of selected infectious diseases (often bats and fruit bats); the clinical symptoms of viral diseases and the most widely used diagnostic methods for the correct identification of the pathogen involved; and a discussion on Japanese encephalitis (JE) as an infectious disease caused by a virus transmitted by blood-sucking arthropods.

Chapter I – Viral hemorrhagic fevers (VHFs) represent a collection of illnesses caused by several distinct viral families. While some types of hemorrhagic fever viruses can cause relatively mild illnesses, many of these viruses cause life-threatening diseases. In general, the term "viral hemorrhagic fever" describes a severe multisystem syndrome. Typical for this syndrome is a systemic damage of vascular system often accompanied by hemorrhages. Nevertheless the bleeding itself is rarely life-threatening. In the autumn and winter of 2014 every day professional and popular press published new information about Ebola outbreak in West Africa. It was not just data related to the number of patients, new recommendations and protocols, information about testing of potential vaccines, but also theoretical works that tried to analyze the situation and data. Authors were trying to answer questions why Ebola virus emerged again in West Africa, and what it meant for the future.

Chapter II – Viral hemorrhagic fever (VHF) disorders represent a group of diseases caused by viruses from several viral families (*Arenaviruses, Filoviruses, Bunyaviruses* and *Flaviviruses*). Such disorders are classified as acute viral febrile diseases characterized by nausea, myalgia and fatigue, with the dominant feature of general alteration of vessel permeability. Symptoms of bleeding, which are usually diffused and present a symptom of general vessel injury rather than a life-threatening condition often occur, particularly in severe cases. Viral hemorrhagic fevers can present as a range of disorders from relatively moderate to human life-threatening conditions with high mortality rates.

Chapter III – Bats and fruit bats belong to animals able to transmit a plenty of different microorganisms as result in infection of domestic animals or humans. It concerns not only viruses or bacteria but fungi and parasite agents too. Although generally the risk of transmission is not so high, it should be considered and it is advisable for humans to handle with such animals in a proper way.

Chapter IV – The New World clade of the *Arenaviridae* family includes several hemorrhagic fever viruses which are important emerging pathogens in South America. The four most significant members of the viral family in this aspect are Junín virus (JUNV), causative agent of the Argentine Hemorrhagic Fever (AHF); Machupo virus (MACV), etiological agent of Bolivian Hemorrhagic Fever (BHF); Guanarito virus (GTOV), which causes Venezuelan Hemorrhagic Fever (VeHF) and Sabiá virus (SABV), causing Brazilian Hemorrhagic Fever (BrHF). Although they are currently constrained to relatively small geographic regions, the global concern regarding these infections is in rise since the outbreak of the Ebola epidemic. Here the authors describe the clinical symptoms of these viral diseases and the most widely used diagnostic methods for the correct identification of the pathogen involved. The analysis of recent epidemiological data in conjunction with climatic and cultural changes shows the imprint of human activity on the environment and can easily be related to the viral emergence.

Chapter V – Japanese encephalitis (JE) is an infectious disease caused by a virus transmitted by blood-sucking arthropods. JE, together with California encephalitis, Saint Louis encephalitis, Central European encephalitis and Russian spring-summer encephalitis, is serious disease affecting the nervous system. After the introduction of universal vaccination against polio, JE is according to the WHO (World Health Organization), worldwide leading disease leading to paretic neuroinfections. It is a vaccine preventable disease typically found in Asia and Western Pacific.

In: Hemorrhagic Fever
Editor: Shirley R. Edwards

ISBN: 978-1-63482-791-1

Chapter I

Viral Hemorrhagic Fevers: Yesterday and Today (Consequences of Ebola Outbreak in West Africa)

V. Bostik[1,*], M. Salavec[2], R. Sleha[1], N. Bostik[1], P. Bostik[1], E. Slehova[3], R. Kukla[3], H. Stritecka[4] and P. Prasil[5]

[1]Faculty of Military Health Sciences, University of Defence, Hradec Kralove, Czech Republic

[2]Department of Dermatovenereology, Charles University Medical School and University Hospital, Hradec Kralove, Czech Republic

[3]Faculty of Chemical-Technology, University of Pardubice, Pardubice, Czech Republic

[4]Department of Military Internal Medicine and Military Hygiene Faculty of Military Health Sciences, University of Defence, Hradec Kralove, Czech Republic

[5]Department of Infectious Diseases, Charles University, Medical School and Faculty Hospital, Hradec Kralove, Czech Republic

[*] Corresponding author: V. Bostik, Faculty of Military Health Sciences, University of Defence, Trebesska 1575, 500 01 Hradec Kralove, Czech Republic. Tel: (420) 973 253 205; E-mail address: vanda.bostikova@unob.cz (Vanda Bostik).

Abstract

Viral hemorrhagic fevers (VHFs) represent a collection of illnesses caused by several distinct viral families. While some types of hemorrhagic fever viruses can cause relatively mild illnesses, many of these viruses cause life-threatening diseases. In general, the term "viral hemorrhagic fever" describes a severe multisystem syndrome. Typical for this syndrome is a systemic damage of vascular system often accompanied by hemorrhages. Nevertheless the bleeding itself is rarely life-threatening.

In the autumn and winter of 2014 every day professional and popular press published new information about Ebola outbreak in West Africa. It was not just data related to the number of patients, new recommendations and protocols, information about testing of potential vaccines, but also theoretical works that tried to analyze the situation and data. Authors were trying to answer questions why Ebola virus emerged again in West Africa, and what it meant for the future.

Introduction

At the time this chapter was written more than 23,900 cases of Ebola virus infection had been reported in West African countries and over 9,700 people already died. Despite of some success due to improvements in the isolation of cases and prevention of the epidemic spread e.g. in Nigeria, the reported number of total cases have been ever increasing [1].

Ebola Virus

VHFs may be caused by viruses from five distinct families of RNA viruses: *Arenaviridae*, *Filoviridae*, *Bunyaviridae*, *Flaviviridae*, and *Rhabdoviridae*. The family *Filoviridae* includes two genera - *Ebolavirus* and *Marburgvirus* [2]. There are five identified Ebola virus species, four of which are known to cause disease in humans: Ebola virus (*Zaire ebolavirus*); Sudan virus (*Sudan ebolavirus*); Taï Forest virus (*Taï Forest ebolavirus*, formerly *Côte d'Ivoire ebolavirus*); and Bundibugyo virus (*Bundibugyo ebolavirus*). The fifth, Reston virus (*Reston ebolavirus*), has caused disease in nonhuman primates, but not in humans.

From molecular genetic analyses we know that the sequence of the Ebola virus strain circulating in this outbreak in west Africa is similar by its sequences to the Zaire strain (ZEBOV), al (though there are with tens of mutations) is circulating in west Africa. The ZEBOV strain was responsible for the first epidemic in Zaire (today Democratic Republic of the Congo) in 1976, when (431 of 602 patients died). Mutations in the sequence of the Ebola virus strain(circulating in west Africa) sequence obviously resulted in decreased numbers of hemorrhagic cases, thus decreasing mortality rate compared to Zaire strain (mortality rate up to 90%). Lower data numbers of hemorrhagic cases and, similar symptoms to some other diseases with, massive occurrence in the area, of such as malaria, typhus fever and cholera, together with a fact, that the outbreak occurred in an area problem was recorded in, where previously not reported Ebola had not been reported before – all this resulted in the delay of correct diagnosis and late detection of this epidemic [3, 4].

Distribution and Reservoirs of VHFs

Causative agents of VHFs are geographically distributed at all settled continents. Natural reservoirs, which were identified only recently, are rodents, fruit bats, ungulate African animals and primates. Humans represent a dead end of the natural transmission chain [5].

Transmission of Ebola Virus

Transmissions in the beginning of epidemic occur by a contact with an infected animal due to scratching or bite, or by consuming an infected meal, especially fruit. Ebola virus specifically is transmitted frequently by infected fruit-bats. These animals frequently only bite into the fruit and contaminate it by saliva containing virus. Infected fruit is then eaten by local natives. Fruit bats are also regarded as favourite delicacy as fresh-caught and dried. About 100,000 fruit bats are sold at markets as food in Ghana in a year [6]. Human to human transmission then continues by a contact with body fluids in consequence. The Ebola virus was detected in blood, breast milk, saliva, vomitus, urine and in genital secretions.

At current state of knowledge it is not possible to anticipate individual cases of infection and predict the development of epidemics [7, 13].

Potential Initiating Factors of the West Africa Ebola Outbreak

One of the opinions indicates that the current outbreak could have been supported or even brought about by changing ecological factors. Countries like Guinea, Liberia or Sierra Leone destroy thousands of hectares of tropical forest for decades due to the mining activities. This changes country climate and draws locals closer to wildlife in order to obtain food by hunting. Time intervals of drought and rainy seasons vary as well as their characters. Such modified climate conditions then support spreading of Ebola virus [8].

According to one of the newer analyses based on ecologic and demographic factors, theoretically fifteen African countries, where virus was mostly never detected, are currently threatened by Ebola virus (Nigeria, Cameroon, Central African Republic, Ghana, Liberia, Sierra Leone, Angola, Tanzania, Togo, Ethiopia, Mosambique, Burundi, Madagaskar, Malawi, Equatorial Guinea [7]).

Population behavior in areas of epidemic spreading also has a significant influence. As one could see at the example of presumptive current epidemic outset, big problems in the infection spreading are generated by local habits, e.g. ritual funerals and other, where a close contact with body fluids of patients and dead occurs [9].

Only targeted and detailed educational training with preventive repressive measures implemented gradually could efficiently help in such cases. Since there is neither a specific drug treatment nor a vaccine available (in spite of currently running clinical trials), such measures are even more important.

Index Case of the Ebola Outbreak in West Africa

On December 26, 2013, two years old boy became sick in Meliandou village in Guinea. He suffered from fever, vomitus, had black stool and died two days later. Fourteen of his relatives and other people preparing his funeral consequently died. At the same time organization called "Doctors Without Borders" was fighting with cholera infection in this area. Specimens were sent to Institute of Pasteur in March 2014 by representatives of this organization. Results confirmed suspected diagnosis of first known Ebola virus occurrence in west Africa [1].

Ebola Virus on the Way – Uncontrolled Epidemic

In Sierra Leone the initial case was successfully managed. The patient was pregnant female with abortus, correctly isolated in governmental hospital in Kailahunu (24. 5. 2014). Unfortunately, the outbreak became uncontrolled with a death of a highly respected healer in the border zone. Hundreds of people from Sierra Leone and neighboring countries took part in a ritual funeral associated with dead body wash-up, touching and embracing a body and farewell kisses. When the now infected funeral guests returned to their homes the virus spread was initiated to distant areas. About 365 subsequent Ebola deaths are closely associated with this funeral. West African statistics attribute a total of 60% share in infection spreading to the ritual funerals [1].

The Medical Care System – New Experiences

Fundamental in pathogenesis of Ebola virus infection is a multi organ system failure. It is therefore necessary to guarantee a high quality medical care due to the absence of both specific antiviral therapy and vaccine. Such medical care is clearly very difficult to provide in poor African countries. Just to compare – seventy medical professionals including laboratory staff cared for one patient with Ebola infection in Emory University Hospital in Atlanta, Georgia, USA. Three nurses took 8 hour shifts in the isolation unit (initially, 12hour shifts were considered, but it was found unrealistic and shifts were shortened on the direct request of the staff). First experience in the successful management of two patients at Emory show a significant importance of a detailed symptomatic therapy with an evaluation of previous health status (immune system, quality of nutrition). The symptomatic treatment includes rehydration with glucose solution and electrolytes (orally, *p.o.*), analgesics, antipyretics, antiemetics, drugs for diarrhoea, sedatives and major tranquilizers, as well as continual blood pressure and oxygen saturation check [10].

The Kaiser Oakland Hospital, the UC San Francisco, the Emory Atlanta, the Rush Chicago, the John Hopkins Baltimore, the Bellevue New York City and 29 other hospital centers across the USA are since December 2014 equipped and ready to take care of patients with a diagnosis of VHF Ebola. Such hospitals became so called Ebola Treatment Centers based on the demographic data analysis. It is known that 80% of travellers from west Africa live in a circle of 160 km of selected hospitals, or in areas surrounding five US international airports (the JFK in New York, the New Jersey Newark Liberty, The Washington Dulles, the Chicago O´Hara and The Hartsfield-Jackson in Atlanta), which are the only airports for controlled landing of flights coming from African areas with outbreak. An activated hospital staff and laboratory compartment are currently trained to diagnose and admit patients in these selected health facilities several hours after landing [1].

Outside the USA, a total of 2,450 US military virologists and microbiologists serve in west Africa in seven large hospital bases. Establishment of such mobile diagnostic labs significantly helped to reduce time between obtaining a specimen to its analysis. In the very beginning of the outbreak it took weeks to obtain the results, due to the distance to the specialized laboratories and their small numbers. Currently results are available in hours, calculated from the time of collecting, which could dramatically improve the chances to save lives.

Laboratory staff speaks about enormous stress, to which they are daily exposed. Each tube means not only number and specimen but is associated with specific human destiny as in case of blood specimen of nine years old Guinean boy. His specimen contained still not observed level of viral load, outside of the usual range 1-10. In this case there was no doubt about further fatal development of the diseases. Sad stories are mercifully replaced by more optimistic ones. Health workers together with natives developed ritual for cured patients, which gives a psychological support to both sides. Every cured patient passes through a nurse /attendant/ lane. They embrace themselves and hand over minor gifts. Every cured patient receives "Ebola Cure Certificate" and brand new clothing and linen [12].

Medical staff continue to learn and train additional necessary safety measures, such as safe handling of medical tools, mutual check of protective suit in a sequence of control steps, disinfection of all material, but they also try make practical life easier by designation of renowned names to laboratory devices like Rambo (specimen analyzer) or Chuck Norris. Such instruments analyze collected material for presence or absence of nucleic acid of Ebola virus and determine viral load parameters in analyzed specimen. A green straight line displayed on the PC monitor means negativity of the specimen. An ascending line indicates positivity and the incline correlates with viral load. All staff in Africa or anywhere in the USA is assigned to these laboratories on the voluntary basis. They know that it is very important to accept any criticism in a positive way and that a mutual check and reminder should be accepted positively and could prevent fatal mistakes [5, 12].

Conclusion

CDC Director in Atlanta Tom Frieden said that the American health system must be activated for possible Ebola management for as long as the virus continues to spread in west Africa.

In Africa, successful cure unfortunately does not lead to permanent solutions of local population problems. The current patients are released from medical centres, but they very often find, that they have nowhere to return. Members of their families are dead or there are only few people surviving. Property of such people had to be burned according to hygienic measures. Survivors are stigmatized by the community, particularly women are often regarded as witches, and they are not able to return to their usual physical labor. They suffer from persistent cephalea, muscle weakness and muscle and back pain. One hundred and seventy died- off farmer families in the food production area of Liberia, in Lofa County, resulted in jeopardy of the food production for the entire country. Use of the entire local capacity and international help to fight Ebola virus infection stopped ongoing health programs to fight malaria and HIV infection.

The Ebola virus has become an unwelcome reminder that, for all its advances, modern medicine has yet to win the war against infectious diseases.

References

[1] www.cdc.gov

[2] Suzuki Y, Gojobori T. The origin and evolution of Ebola and Marburg viruses. *Mol Biol Evol.*1997;14: 800 - 806.

[3] Center for disease control and prevention. Chronology of Ebola hemorrhagic fever outbreaks. Accessed: August 2014. Available from: http://www. cdc.gov/vhf/ebola/resources/outbreak-table.html.

[4] Pigott DM, Golding N, Mylne A, et al. Mapping the zoonotic niche of Ebola virus disease in Africa. *eLife* 2014;3:e04395. DOI: 10.7554/eLife.04395.

[5] Sanchez A, Ksiazek TG, Rollin PE, et al. Reemergence of Ebola virus in Africa. *Emerg Infect Dis.* 1995; 1: 96-97.

[6] Pourrut X, Souris M, Towner JS, et al. Large serological survey showing cocirculation of Ebola and Marburg viruses in Gabonese bat population, and a high seroprevalence of both viruses in *Rousettus aegyptiacus. BMC Infect Dis.* 2009; 9:159.

[7] Chan M. Ebola virus disease in West Africa - no early end to the outbreak. *The New England Journal of Medicine.* 2014. doi: 10.156/NEJMp1409859.

[8] Brashares JS, Golden CD, Weinbaum KZ, Barrett CB, Okello GV. Economic and geographic drivers of wildlife consumption in rural Africa. *Proceedings of the National Academy of Sciences of USA.* 2011;108:13931–6. doi: 10.1073/pnas.1011526108.

[9] Simini F, Maritan A, Neda Z. Human mobility in a continuum approach. 2013. *PLOS ONE* 8:e60069. doi: 10.1371/ journal.pone.0060069.

[10] Briand S, Bertherat E, Cox P, Formenty P, Kieny MP, Myhre JK, et al. The international Ebola emergency. *The New England Journal of Medicine* 2014. doi: 10.1056/NEJMp1409858.

[11] Appleton BR, McKenzie JA, Christidis L. Molecular systematice and biogeography of the bent-wing bat complex *Miniopterus schreibersii* (Kuhl, 1817) (Chiroptera: Vespertilionidae). *Mol Phylogenet Evol.* 2004; 31: 431-439.

[12] Leroy EM, Kumulungui B, Pourrut X, et al. Fruit bats as reservoirs of Ebola virus. *Nature* 438: 575-576 (2005).

[13] EMORY Medicine, special issue. 2014, 1 -35.

In: Hemorrhagic Fever
Editor: Shirley R. Edwards

ISBN: 978-1-63482-791-1

Chapter II

Selected Viral Hemorrhagic Fevers: A Lot of Questions, Few Answers

V. Bostik[1,*], M. Salavec[2], P. Prasil[3] and P. Bostik[1]

[1]Faculty of Military Health Sciences,
University of Hradec Kralove, Czech Republic
[2]Department of Dermatovenerology,
Charles University Medical School and University Hospital,
Hradec Kralove, Czech Republic
[3]Department of Infectious Diseases, Charles University,
Medical School and Faculty Hospital, Hradec Kralove, Czech Republic

Abstract

Viral hemorrhagic fever (VHF) disorders represent a group of diseases caused by viruses from several viral families (*Arenaviruses, Filoviruses, Bunyaviruses* and *Flaviviruses*). Such disorders are classified as acute viral febrile diseases characterized by nausea, myalgia and fatigue, with the dominant feature of general alteration of vessel

* Corresponding author: V. Bostik, Faculty of Military Health Sciences, University of Defence, Trebesska 1575, 500 01 Hradec Kralove, Czech Republic. Tel: (420) 973 253 205, E-mail address: vanda.bostikova@unob.cz (Vanda Bostik).

permeability. Symptoms of bleeding, which are usually diffused and present a symptom of general vessel injury rather than a life-threatening condition often occur, particularly in severe cases. Viral hemorrhagic fevers can present as a range of disorders from relatively moderate to human life-threatening conditions with high mortality rates.

Introduction

Having a look into the history of infectious diseases, we can characterize individual centuries in terms of a particular disease which plagued people of that time: the 12th century was the century of variola, the 13th century we can call the century of leprosy, the 14th century was the century of plague and we associate the 15th century with syphilis. In the 16th century, civilization suffered from dysentery and during the 17th century, people died of tuberculosis. In the 18th century, typhoid fever plagued humanity and in the 19th century, they died because of cholera. We will not be wrong in choosing HIV/AIDS as the characteristic disease for the 20th century. It is not easy to predict the major disease for the 21st century in 2015, but speculation allows us to consider viral hemorrhagic fevers (VHF).

Rapid and widely available intercontinental travel leading to an accelerated migration of large numbers of people are factors that opened new possibilities of spreading viruses and associated infectious diseases to other geographical areas.

The most frequently imported infection in recent years worldwide is malaria. The prime example is the so-called “airport form”, which typically develops in people living close to large airports as seen in England, France, and Madeira. Another purely air-travel imported disease over the last few years is the West Nile virus (WNV) infection, which traveled from the African continent to the Eastern U.S. and gradually spread along the East Coast all the way to the West Coast of the United States.

In response to these developments, epidemiologic measures were introduced, which included a disinfection of aircraft coming from subtropical and tropical areas. However, transmission of many of these newly imported diseases including those mentioned above involves an important element—the vector. In most of these cases, various species of mosquitoes serve as vectors between natural viral reservoirs and humans. The European continent in recent years has begun to be threatened by invasive mosquito species previously not found there, such as *Aedes albopictus*. These insects find their way to the area by, for example, importation of plants from endemic areas. The previous notion of the inability of these invasive species to cope with colder European climate has not been confirmed so far. The usual breeding habitats of these insects, such as used tyres stored outdoors with water, are available in the "new" countries as well.

Several reports have emerged recently describing findings of these insects in the Danube Delta in Romania, Albania, Sicily, Sardinia, Corsica, Greece, Madeira, San Marino, Vatican City and in Dutch green- houses. Seventeen nymphs of *Aedes albopictus* species were identified in South Moravia in the Czech Republic recently [1]. This species is known as the vector for dengue and chikungunya viruses. This particular species will likely have problems with acclimatization, since it does not tolerate low temperatures. The related *Aedes japonicus* species - a vector for WNV, which tolerates a wide range of temperatures, was identified in Belgium, France and in the Rhine valley in Germany. Another WNV vector, *Aedes atropalpus*, which was typical for North America and thus adapted for colder climate, has been discovered in Italy, France and the Netherlands. *Aedes triseriatus* species, the vector for the La Crosse virus group causing encephalitis, has been detected in France. This is only a small example of about 100 estimated invasive mosquito species [2, 3]. Due to this emerging situation, several countries such as France and Italy, are developed a monitoring system which should keep track of these newly appearing invasive mosquito species.

Viral Hemorrhagic Fever Diseases

Viral hemorrhagic fevers constitute a group of infectious diseases characterized by a severe symptomatology, which includes bleeding and high mortality rate. They are typically distributed in certain geographic areas, but they are not common in Europe, where the individual cases usually represent imported infections. In such cases, it is quite often difficult to make a rapid diagnosis and introduce epidemiological measures, thus it is helpful to perform the risk estimation, which reflects a likelihood that the particular patient acquired the VHF during their previous travel. The minimal risk situations are those, when a person in consideration did not visit the endemic area of VHF, or more than 21 days passed between the visit and first health problems. The moderate risk is characterized by the travel of the patient to the endemic area within the 21 days period before the disease onset, but with no contact with people suffering from VHF. The high risk is determined, when the person was present in the risk area within 3 weeks before the onset of symptoms and by contact lasting more than 4 hours in household with VHF patient.

The VHF diseases are typically characterized by febrile states associated with bleeding and high mortality rates [4]. Causative agents of these infectious diseases group are RNA viruses encapsulated by lipid membrane. These viruses belong to four different virus families: *Arenaviridae, Flaviviridae, Filoviridae* and *Bunyaviridae*. This large diversity of the potential causative viruses contributes to the diversity of symptomatology of the VHF diseases and to difficulties to specify in details their common symptoms [5, 6].

Arenaviridae genus includes African Lassa virus causing Lassa fever and South American viruses Junin, Machupo, Guanarito and Sabia, which cause Bolivian, Argentine, Venezuela and Brazil hemorrhagic fever.

The Lassa virus is a RNA virus formed by 2 linear RNA segments, of 7 200 and 3 400 nt in length, which are encapsulated by a lipid membrane. It received its name after the city of Lassa in Nigeria, where the disease first occurred in 1969. The course of the infection can range from asymptomatic to severe, which can result in patient's death due to the multiple organ failure.. The typical incubation period ranges between 5 – 21 days. The symptomatic patients suffer from high fever, headache, myalgia, cough, laryngitis, vomitus and diarrhea. Conjunctivitis could also develop, as well as the petechial rash on the chest, hands and face.. In 20% of the patients low blood pressure levels due to epistaxis, gingival and rectal bleeding are present. Encephalitis and meningitis could also develop. In pregnant women infected during 3rd trimester spontaneous abort can occur, which is lethal for the fetus in 100% and for mother in about 30% of cases. The diagnosis of Lassa fever can be confirmed by Reverse Transcriptase- Polymerase Chain Reaction (RT PCR), serologically by Enzyme-linked immunosorbent assay (ELISA) test or by virus isolation. The antiviral therapy by ribavirin reduces mortality from 55% to 5%. Other therapeutic measures include fluid management - replenishment and management of patient in shock. The vector of the virus is a rodent – rat living in west and middle Africa close to human residences. Unfortunately these rats are regarded as a delicacy for natives and it is often consumed. Thus an important preventive measure is an education about the dangers associated with such practices. Infection can also be transmitted by a contact with infected animal excrements, urine and saliva through minor skin defects, or by aerosol inhalation of infected aerosols. The occurrence of Lassa virus was also suspected in Congo, Mali and in Senegal. Estimated 5000 individuals die annually of Lassa virus infection worldwide [7, 8].

The Junin virus, which causes the Argentinian hemorrhagic fever, was first isolated in 1958. It is frequently classified as a New World virus due to its geographical occurrence. Symptoms of the disease include typically low fever, chills, headache, myalgia, petechial on face, neck and chest areas, conjunctivitis, gingival bleeding, hand tremor and general stupor. Neurologic symptoms, shock, blood expectoration, blood in urine and stool and infinite" menstruation period develop in 30% of the patients. Secondary bacterial infections could develop as complications. The main diagnostic test is serology performed by ELISA. Rodents serve both as vectors and reservoirs of infection. Transmission to humans occurs by inhalation of the dust contaminated by urine, excrements, saliva and blood, or through a minor skin trauma serving as the port of entry for viral aerosol. For the treatment an immune serum obtained from convalescent patients is used. A safe and efficient live attenuated vaccine is available as a preventive measure, which has been already administered to about 150 000 humans and which has shown a protective effect in the Bolivian hemorrhagic fever in animal experiments as well [5, 6].

The Machupo virus, another New World virus, is a causative agent of the Bolivian hemorrhagic fever. After 7-14 days of incubation rapidly increasing fever, headache, myalgia, arthralgia, malaise, skin paresthesias, neurologic and hemorrhagic symptoms develop in infected individuals. In severe cases skin petechial, face edema, epistaxis, gingival and vaginal bleeding leading to a shock with hand tremors develop eventually leading to the coma. Rodents, again, serve as the reservoirs of the virus and transmission by mechanisms similar to the Junin virus has been proven. In 1994, however, six fatal cases where human to human transmission occurred within one family in Magdalena city in Bolivia were described [5, 6].

Flaviridae family is represented by Omsk hemorrhagic fever virus (middle Asia), Kyasanur forest fever virus (India), virus of yellow fever (Africa, South America) and Dengue virus (Africa, Asia, North and South America, Pacific region) [9].

The Omsk hemorrhagic fever (OHF) is caused by a virus with linear RNA of 10 400 nt size length. Usually two viral strains are described – Kubrin and Bogulovovska strains. Experimental work with this virus has to be performed in the highest Biosafety level laboratory - BSL 4. This virus is not associated with neurological involvement. Incubation period ranges between 2 and 10 days. Clinical presentations include biphasic fever, headache, cough, dehydration, conjunctivitis, papulovesicular lesions on soft palate and typical splenomegaly. Mortality rate reaches 3%. Serologic ELISA test and virus isolation confirm the diagnosis. Tick of *Dermacentor* genus is the vector of the disease, while the musk-rat, water-rat, amphibians and reptiles in endemic areas (middle Siberia, Omsk and Novosibirsk region) are reservoirs. Virus was even successfully isolated from water where the infected animals were living, which suggests that it is a very stable virus. Human infections caused by an ingestion of milk from infected goats and sheep, which were in contact with dead animals have been proven. Musk-rat hunters are at risk of infections acquired from dead animals, however tick borne infection was frequently confirmed as well. Seven infections were detected in 1998 in Novosibirsk region, one of which resulted in death. The regular use of repellents is recommended as the preventive measure in the endemic areas. Treatment is based on supportive and symptomatic care represented mainly by the fluid replenishment. According to published results, the vaccine against tick encephalitis induces some immunity against OHF as well [5, 6].

Kyasanur forest fever. Causative viral agent was successfully isolated from infected monkey in the Kyanasur forest in India (endemic area) in 1957, but it has been recently isolated also in Saudi Arabia. Small rodents, bats and monkeys represent the reservoirs and ticks transmit this virus also to goat, sheep and cattle. We still have no evidence on transmission by the unpasteurized milk to humans. In humans, fever, headache, myalgia, cough, dehydration, nausea and bleeding typically develop after 3 to 8 days of incubation period [5, 6].

Yellow fever. This diseases is caused by a virus containing linear RNA of 10 862 nt length with seven known genotypes. Phylogenetic studies showed, that this virus is 3 000 years old. The disease originated in Africa and Spanish conquerors imported the virus to the Central and South Americas. First reports of the disease were described in the diaries of Spanish catholic missionaries living among Mayo population in the first half of the 17th century. The virus was first isolated from an infected man in Ghana in 1972 (Asabi strain prototype). After the incubation period of 3 – 6 days the infection presents with fever, chill, myalgia, headache, vomitus and lower abdominal pain. Jaundice develops in patients and multi organ failure involving liver, kidney and subsequent shock can develop. RT-PCR and ELISA tests are carried out to confirm diagnosis. The virus circulates among the hosts in two different cycles - sylvatic (rural) and urban.

A great yellow fever epidemics occurred in 1960 in Ethiopia with some 30 000 individuals being infected. In 1978 Gambia reported 8 400 patients with 1 600 cases resulting in death. Nigeria suffered from yellow fever epidemics in 1987, where 565 cases out of 1 450 infected patients were lethal. Other local epidemics in Bolivia, Brasilia, Colombia, Peru, Cameroon, Mali, and Senegal and in Togo were reported in 2007. Highly reliable vaccine is available for this disease based on the attenuated strain 17D, which is effective against all known genotypes of this virus. It cannot be administered in risk groups, i.e. in children, in individuals with immunodeficiency and egg allergy patients [5, 6].

Dengue. Dengue epidemics in Philippines and in Thailand in the 50´s of the last century raised attention to the virus occurring in 4 serologic types, which contains linear RNA 10 200 long. A successful cure of the infection caused by one of the serotypes does not mean immunity against the other serologic types. Dengue can thus affect one individual repeatedly and the re-infections are caused by different serotypes. Moreover, the course of the infection is predetermined by the sequence of the individual serotypes, which induce the re-infection in one individual. Both older children and adults are involved. Clinically the infection presents by a mild or classical fever, and in the most severe cases as a life-threatening hemorrhagic fever. Humans are infected by mosquitoes and after 4-7 days fever of 38 ^{o} C to 41° C develops with headache, myalgia, arthralgia, vomitus and photophobia. Then the temperature decreases for about 24 hours, but it can recur with the development of skin erythema, maculopapular rash and petechiae. Diagnosis is confirmed by RT-PCR and serologic ELISA test. Dengue is also circulates in two cycles - sylvatic form (associated with monkeys and mosquito species) and urban form (humans and mosquito species). Transovarial type of transmission of the virus in mosquitoes was described, as well as the transmission by sexual intercourse and blood – transfusion in humans. Humans and primates are the main viral reservoir. Dengue occurs in tropical and subtropical areas in all regions, where mosquito species are present. It seems that boat travel in the 18th and in 19th century contributed to worldwide virus spreading in all affected regions. Similarly, the expansion of business activities led to the spread throughout the Southeast Asia after WWII. Treatment is still largely based on supportive measures including the administration of antipyretics, plasma, blood transfusions and anti-shock treatment. Therefore the prevention is important – regular use of insecticides, mosquito net, slop desiccation and still waters and fenland (essential for mosquito survival) elimination. It is indicated that up to 40% of world population live in areas at risk of dengue infection [5, 6, and 9].

Filoviridae family includes Ebola and Marburg viruses. These RNA viruses (19000 nt) are typical for Africa and west parts of the Pacific region [9, 11].

While the pathogenesis of many VHFs remains unknown, the current model of Ebola virus (EV) infection depicts the Ebola virus dissemination from an infection site (minor trauma) to regional lymph nodes and then to liver and spleen. Though EV does not infect lymphocytes, a rapid decline of lymphocyte counts due to apoptosis is the main symptom of the disease. It is not possible to exclude direct interaction of lymphocytes with viral proteins as one of the reasons for their destruction, but the rapid depletion is probably based on a combination of dendritic cell dysfunction and release of soluble monocyte and macrophage derived mediators [6].

Incubation period ranges between 3-21 days and subsequent symptoms include headache, myalgia, abdominal pain, vomitus, watery or bloody diarrhea, skin rash, hemorrhage, dehydration, and shock and multi organ failure. In surviving patients the convalescent phase takes a long course. Transmissions due to close contacts with blood, secrets or tissue of infected individuals or primates (gorillas and chimpanzees) were reported. Reservoir of EV was elusive for a long time. First in association with the EV epidemic in Congo in 2009, fruit bats were recognized as reservoirs for Ebola and Marburg viruses. Epidemics occurred unpredictably from time to time mainly in Congo, Sudan, Gabon, Republic of South Africa, Ivory Coast, Uganda and Philippines. EV type Reston was detected in swine in conjunction with EV specific antibodies in farmer's serum in 2008. None of the known antiviral agents including ribavirin are efficient in Ebola infection. Fears of EV are so huge that three Japanese airlines refused to transport monkey deliveries [11, 12, and 13].

Marburg virus got his name after the German city of Marburg, where infections originating from African green monkeys imported from Uganda occurred. Lab worker, who took care of the monkeys and manipulated with monkey tissue samples was infected first. Thirty-one infected individuals, out of whom 25 primary and 6 secondary infections were reported. Seven primary infections resulted in death. Another epidemics in the cities of Frankfurt and Belgrade occurred 1967.

Incubation period ranges between 3-9 days. Fever, headache, myalgia, abdominal pain, nausea, vomitus, diarrhea, maculopapular rash, lethargy, cough, conjunctivitis and photophobia then appear, and hemorrhage, gastrointestinal, vaginal, gingival bleeding and shock develop in about 45% of cases. Mortality rate ranges between 25 and 90%. Serologic ELISA tests and RT-PCR or virus isolation are laboratory methods used to confirm the diagnosis.

Marburg virus is transmitted by blood and secrets of infected humans or animals, particularly monkeys. Fruit bats serve as virus reservoirs. Transmission by aerosols has not been proven in nature yet. Nosocomial and laboratory infections have been reported. Epidemics occur most frequently in Zimbabwe, Republic of South Africa, Kenya, Congo, and Angola and in Uganda. The big epidemic was described in 2004-2005 in Angola, where 356 individuals out of 422 involved died of Marburg infection.

Limited number of therapeutical approaches are available – rehydration, respiratory supportive measures and blood transfusions. Preventive measures are focused on the education of locals [13, 23].

Crimean-Congo hemorrhagic fever (Africa, Eastern Europe, middle Asia), Rift Valley fever (Africa, the Middle East) and Hantaan viruses (Asia, Africa, the Balkan Peninsula) are members of the *Bunyaviridae* family [14].

Rift Valley Fever Virus. The virus was first identified in 1931 during an investigation of an epidemic among sheep on a farm in the Rift Valley of Kenya. It is a RNA virus organized into 3 linear segments. Incubation period is 2-5 days. Infected either experience no detectable symptoms or develop a mild form of the disease characterized by sudden onset of flu-like fever, muscle pain, joint pain, myalgia, headache and vomitus. The disease often cures spontaneously after one week. About one fifth of patients suffer from ophthalmologic problems including temporary blindness and more severe symptoms, such as meningoencephalitis, hallucinations, blood emesis and bleeding (e.g. at injection site) in the hemorrhagic form. Mortality in such severe cases reaches 50%. Several mosquito species serve as vectors for the virus, while sheep, cattle, goats, camels and rodents are known reservoirs. The infection can also occur by a direct contact with an infected animal, infected animal blood or tissue fluids. RT-PCR assay and virus isolation by cell culture are the most frequently used methods for the diagnosis. Inactivated vaccine was tested in veterinarians and in laboratory staff, but it is commercially unavailable. Only supporting measures including artificial ventilation and blood transfusion are available for treatment. The first epidemic outside of the African continent was reported in Saudi Arabia and Yemen in 2000, In association with these epidemics first speculations occurred on when this infection arrives in Europe and how well prepared appropriate measures are [6, 15].

Hantaviruses. These viruses constitute 2 large groups – so called Old world viruses including Hantaan River, Dobrava-Belgrade, Soul, Puumala, Tobetsu, and Topografov, Tula species which cause diseases characterized by the hemorrhagic fever with renal syndrome or nephropathy (HFRS). The second group called New Word viruses includes the following virus species – Prospect Hill, Isla Vista, Leaky, Blue River, Black Creek Canal, which cause Hantavirus pulmonary syndrome (HPS). Viral genome is organized into three linear segments encapsulated by lipid membrane.

Typical symptoms in HFRS include fever, headache, myalgia, chills, cough, vomiting and renal insufficiency, as well as mild nasal, vaginal and gastrointestinal hemorrhage.

Some of the virus species, such as Tula, are almost non-pathogenic, while others show varying mortality rates – Dobrava 5-35%, Soul 1%.

Prodromal symptoms of HPS include flu-like symptoms such as fever, cough, myalgia, headache, and lethargy. The full-blown disease is characterized by a sudden onset of dyspnea with rapidly evolving pulmonary edema that is often fatal due to shock and heart failure due to pulmonary vessel system hypertension. The fatality rate reaches 40 – 60 %.

ELISA, RT-PCR, immunofluorescence tests and virus isolation using cell culture are indicated. Each virus species has its individual vector – a rodent species specific for the given geographical area. Transmission to humans occurs by contact with rodents or their urine, excrements, saliva, aerosol inhalation and by rodent bites. Typical is inhalation of aerosol containing dust contaminated with dried rodent excreta in field workers. Human to human transmission was proven in Argentina. Supportive care is important, dialysis and ribavirin introduced early during the disease course were shown to reduce the mortality rate and length of treatment. Recurrent infections were recorded in Brasilia in the 1993-2007 period and in Serbia, Montenegro and Croatia in 2002 [16, 17].

Conclusion

It is almost impossible to predict viral hemorrhagic fever epidemic. Viral hemorrhagic fevers typically occur sporadically or in local epidemics. Just in the second half of the year 2012, three epidemics were reported in Africa: on July 28^{th,} Uganda reported an epidemic of Ebola, where 24 individuals were infected and 17 cases were fatal; on October 27th, the Congo reported an Ebola infection of 35 people, 24 cases resulting in death. And, finally, on November 8th, 17 cases of Marburg VHF were reported in Uganda and 9 patients died [5, 18].

Supportive care to keep basic life processes is the main therapeutic approach. It is important to ensure sufficient hydration, blood volume, to control mineral levels, to introduce anti-shock measures and to use artificial ventilation if indicated. In some cases ribavirin, classified as ribonucleic analogue, shows efficacy [20, 21].

In our geographical latitude, diagnosis of imported infections could present a problem. It is due to the minimal experience and due to atypical courses of such viral infections in local population compared to the usually typical clinical presentation in natives in endemic areas.

Difficulties in experimental work due to high infectivity and pathogenicity of these viruses present another complication. This slows research leading to the data on pathogenesis of VHF important for the development of new therapeutic approaches and new drug development research. All manipulation with such viruses must be performed at BSL-4 or BSL-3 level. These are the highest levels of bio-containment, which provide safety for both the laboratory staff and the environment. Handling of these viruses requires laboratory personnel with a special training, (including psychological) and special laboratory equipment, such as sealed rooms, sealed containers, positive pressure personnel suits with an individual air supply, permanent 24-hours movement monitoring system and others. There is a limited number of existing BSL-4 facilities with the appropriate equipment and experienced laboratory staff worldwide. Even at BSL-4 facilities, experimental work and research are significantly time-constrained. The time allowed for the work in special suits is relatively short, which limits types of experimental work that can be performed.

Research focused on the vaccine development is thus a priority. The classical methods of vaccines based on inactivated virus failed. Preferred efforts are now focused on genetic engineering. The NIAID program is developing Ebola vaccine based on an attenuated vesicular stomatitis virus (VSV) containing sequences coding for Ebola specific protein. It is a recombinant vector vaccine where viral vector expresses epitopes of the pathogen and stimulates immune system of vaccinated individuals. Tests with experimental vaccine proved an efficacy in primates. The Lassa virus vaccine has been developed on similar principles. Again it is attenuated recombinant VSV expressing the Lassa virus glycoprotein. A single dose of this vaccine administered *i.m.* successfully protected primates in a study. Nasal spray against Ebola has been tested using a recombinant vaccine based on human parainfluenza virus type 3. This experimental vaccine induced strong immune response in guinea pigs and monkeys [12, 26, and 27].

Due to the absence of both specific protection and treatment, preventive measures focused to avoid contact with sources of infection remain the most important. It is prerequisite to know and trace endemic occurrence areas and, if possible, avoid them. Mosquito and tick protection plays an important role (insecticides, repellents, and mosquito and window nets), as well as the control of the rodent population control.

Training of health care personnel, safety guidelines for manipulation with contaminated material, specimen handling and patient isolation measures are all very important. Functioning of hospital departments intended for VHF patients should be under a special regulations control. The facilities themselves are have to be set up differently compared to common infectious department. Some of the characteristics include negative air pressure, chemical toilets, disinfection of all body excrements, sterilization and incineration of the used material, transportation of clinical samples in duplicated package protection by staff using respirators, eye protection and double gloves, single bed rooms with single entrance through corridor, air circulation through HePa filters, germicidal detergents of 0,5% sodium hypochlorite type, 2% glutaraldehyde and others [25, 27, 30, 31].

Fast and correct diagnosis is extremely important in VHF and should be supported by high-quality lab tests primarily based on molecular genetic methods (PCR, sequencing). Even in Europe and North America, which do not represent endemic areas for VHF, the surveillance and education needs to be at a sufficient level. This is supported by a recent experience with imported VHF cases in these continents and also a recent information about first filovirus with natural occurrence in Europe. It is Ebola-like filovirus called after site of detection – Lloviu virus. Its sequence is in 73.3% identical to Ebola-Zaire sequence and was isolated from dead bats from Cueva del Lloviu cave in southern Spain [22]. The potential for use of VHF as bioterror agents presents another potential danger in virtually any part of the world.

References

[1] Sebesta O., et al.2012. An invasive mosquito species *Aedes albopictus* found in the Moravia. Eurosurveillance, ECDC, no.17, www.eurosurveillance.org/viewarticle.aspx?articleId=20301.

[2] Hoogstraal H. 1979. The epidemiology of tick bone CCHF in Asia, Europe, and Africa. JMedEntomol, no.15, 307-417.

[3] WHO. Cairo.Viral hemorrhagic fever. 2011. Available from: http://www.who.int/mediacentre/factsheets/fs208/en/index.html

[4] Peters C.J., et al.1996. Patients infected with high-hazard viruses: scientific basis for infection controls. *Arch. Virol. Suppl.* no.11, 141 – 168.

[5] Marty A.M., et al. 2006.Viral hemorrhagic fevers. *Clin. Lab. Med.* no.26, 345 – 386.

[6] Peters C.J.2006. Overview of viral hemorrhagic fevers. In: Guerrant R.L., Walker D.H., Weller P.F.: Tropical infectious diseases: principles, pathogens and practice. Philadelphia: Churchill Livingstone.756 – 761.

[7] McCormik J.B. 2002. Lassa fever. *Curr.Top Microbiol. Immunol.* no. 262, 75 – 109.

[8] Monath T.P. 1974.Lassa virus isolation *from Mastomys natalensis* rodents during an epidemic in Sierra Leone. Science. no.185, 263-265.

[9] Guerrant R.L.2006.Tropical infectious diseases: principles, pathogens and practice. Philadelphia: Churchill Livingstone, 756 – 761.

[10] Mupapa K. 1999. Treatment of Ebola hemorrhagic fever with blood tramsfusion from convalescent patients. *J. Infect. Dis*.no. 1, S18 – S 23.

[11] Khan A.S. 2009. A new twist for Ebola: Reston-infected pigs in the Philippines. Public Health Matters. http://www.cdc.gov/nczved/blog/2009/01/05/ebola-reston.html

[12] Jones S.M., et al. 2005. Live attenuated recombinant vaccine protects nonhuman primates against Ebola and Marburg viruses. *Nat.Med.* no. 11(7), 786 – 790.

[13] Leffel E. K., et al. 2004. Marburg and Ebola viruses as aerosol threats. *Biosec. Bioterr.: Biodefense Strat. Pract. Sci. no.* 2(3), 1 – 6.

[14] Ozkurt Z., et al. 2006. Crimean-Congo hemorrhagic fever in Eastern Turkey: clinical features, risk factors and efficacy of ribavirin therapy. *J. Infect. no.* 52, 207 – 215.

[15] Lacy M.D., et al. 1996. Viral hemorrhagic fever. *Adv Pediatr Infect Dis.* no.12, 21-53.

[16] Vapalahti O., et al. 2003.Hantavirus infections in Europe. *Lancet Infect. Dis*. no.3, 653 – 661.

[17] Pejcoch M. 2003.Hantaviruses and their infections. KMIL. no.1(9), 4 – 11.

[18] Khan A.S. 1998. Filoviral haemorrhagic fevers. *Br. Med. Bull.* no. 54 (3), 675-692.

[19] Lub M., et al. 1995. Clinical-virusological characteristics of disease in monkeys in infected with the Marburg virus by an airborne route. *Vopr. Virusol.* No. 40(3), 119 – 121.
[20] Haas W.H., et al. 2003.Imported Lassa and management of contact persons. *Clin. Infect. Dis*. no. 36(10), 1254 -1258.
[21] Demby A.H., et al. 1994.. Early diagnosis of Lassa fever by reverse transcription PCR. *J. Clin. Microbiol*. no.32(12), 2898-2903.
[22] Splino M., et al. 2012. Ebola virus. Vakcinologie. no.2, 80-81.
[23] Bausch D.G., et al. 2003. Risk factor for Marburg HF, Congo. Emerg Infect Dis.no. 9, 1531-1537.
[24] Osterholm M.T., et al. 2002): Hemorrhagic fever viruses as biological weapons. Medical and Public Health Managment. *J. Am. Med. Ass.* no.287, 2391-2405.
[25] CDC. 1988. Management of patients with suspected viral hemorrhagic fever. Morb. Mort. Wk. Rep.37(S-3). 16s. http://www.cdc.gov/mmwr/preview/mmwrhtml/00037085.htm
[26] Geisbert T.W., et al. 2002. Evaluation in nonhuman primates of vaccines against Ebola virus. *Emerg. Infect. Dis.*no. 8, 503 – 507.
[27] WHO. 2009. Ebola Reston found in domestic pigs in the Philippines. Frequently asked questions about Ebola Reston virus and human health. http://www.wpro.who.int/health_topics/ebola_reston/EbolaReston_FAQ.htm
[28] WHO. Crimean-Congo hemorrhagic fever. New Delhi: World Health Organization, SEARO; 2011. http://www.who.int/linkfiles/Communicable_Diseases_Surveillance_and_response_CCHF_Fact_Sheet_SEARO.pdf
[29] Swanepol R., et al.1996. Experimental inoculation of plants and animals with Ebola virus. *Emerg. Infect*. Dis.no. 2, 321 - 325.
[30] CDC.1988. Management of patients with suspected VHF.MMWR.no.37, str.1-16.
[31] Borio L., et al.2002. Medical and public health management. *JAMA*. No.287, 2391-405.

In: Hemorrhagic Fever
Editor: Shirley R. Edwards

ISBN: 978-1-63482-791-1

Chapter III

The Characteristics of Bats and Fruit Bats as Reservoirs of Selected Infectious Diseases with Emphasis on Viral Hemorrhagic Fevers

V. Bostik[1,*], M. Salavec[2], R. Sleha[1], N. Bostik[1], E. Slehova[3], R. Kukla[3] and P. Prasil[4]

[1]Faculty of Military Health Sciences, University of Defence, Hradec Kralove, Czech Republic

[2]Department of Dermatovenereology, Charles University Medical School and University Hospital, Hradec Kralove, Czech Republic

[3]Faculty of Chemical-Technology, University of Pardubice, Pardubice, Czech Republic

[4]Department of Infectious Diseases, Charles University, Medical School and Faculty Hospital, Hradec Kralove, Czech Republic

---

[*] Corresponding author: V. Bostik, Faculty of Military Health Sciences, University of Defence, Trebesska 1575, 500 01 Hradec Kralove, Czech Republic. Tel: (420) 973 253 205. E-mail address: vanda.bostikova@unob.cz (Vanda Bostik).

Abstract

Bats and fruit bats belong to animals able to transmit a plenty of different microorganisms as result in infection of domestic animals or humans. It concerns not only viruses or bacteria but fungi and parasite agents too. Although generally the risk of transmission is not so high, it should be considered and it is advisable for humans to handle with such animals in a proper way.

Bats and Fruit Bats Characteristics

Bats (*Microchiroptera*) and fruit bats (*Megachiroptera*) belong mammalian genus (*Mammalia*), of the order Chiroptera (*Chiroptera,* from the *Greek* χείρ - *cheir*, "hand" and πτερόν - *pteron*, "wing"). They are the only mammalian capable of flying what resulted in cosmopolitan distribution with centre of diversity in tropical regions where there is a higher concentration compared to temperate zone [1].

They developed flying membranes between fingers of upper extremities and another membrane between lower extremities and tail. They orientate oneself due to echolocation. Bat echolocation is a perceptual system where ultrasonic sounds are emitted specifically to produce echoes. By comparing the outgoing pulse with the returning echoes, the brain and auditory nervous system can produce detailed images of the bat's surroundings. This allows bats to detect, localize, and even classify their prey in complete darkness. In addition to echolocating prey, bat ears are sensitive to the fluttering of moth wings, the sounds produced by *tymbalate* insects, and the movement of ground-dwelling prey, such as centipedes, earwigs, etc. Most bats are nocturnal creatures.

The majority of food consumed by bats includes insects, fruits and flower nectar, vertebrates and blood. Compared to representative of the same order, subfamily vampire bats (*Desmodontinae)* are characterized by hematophagy – entirely feeding on warm-blooded animals. These mammalians in Latin and in South America are in that geographical altitude regarded as significant reservoir of rabies [1, 2, 3, 4].

Male and female bats are living in separate groups for most of the year. Female bats manage to preserve sperm in reproductive organs for several months after mating till spring months until eggs fertilization takes part. Gestation period takes two to three months and majority of bat species deliver one, rarely more newborns. Female bats companion with young forming so called summer colonies during summer in temperate zones. Their daylight hours are spent grooming and sleeping in house attics and in tree cavities. Bats could *migrate* hundreds of miles to winter hibernation dens, some pass into *torpor* in cold weather, rousing and feeding when warm weather allows for insects to be active and others retreat to caves for winter and *hibernate* while slowing metabolic processes for six months. Their temperature decreases to 2° C.

The *Chiroptera* order presents 20% of diversity of all mammalian sorts. It is the most diversified and the most widespread order found at all continents except of Antarctica. This and their other characteristics like feed sort, their population structure in multi-thousand colonies, flying ability, seasonal migration to far distance, daily movement figure, torpor and hibernation, lifetime significantly promote zoonotic host role for broad spectrum of antimicrobial agents able to experience so called spill over, i.e. to cross interspecific borders and contaminate domestic and wild animals as well as human individuals [1, 5, 6, 7].

Number of viruses have been detected in chiroptera to the present. Sixty six viruses were identified in 74 different *Chiroptera* species. Arthropoda strains are usually responsible for infection [8]. Frequently it is not clear whether *Chiroptera* are this important viral reservoir. For instance virus Chikungunya or Sindbis of Alphaviruses family (*Togaviridae* tribe), Carey Island virus of Flavivirus family (*Flaviviridae* tribe), Japan encephalitis virus, Jugra virus, Kyasanur forest virus or Rio Bravo virus, further Saint Louis encephalitis virus, Saboya virus, Sokulu and Yokose viruses were reported. From Bunyavirus family (*Bunyaviridae* tribe) Catu virus, Guama virus, Nepuyo virus are listed as Rift Valley fever virus or Toscana virus of Phlebovirus family (*Bunyaviridae* tribe), Ife virus, Japanaut virus and Fomede virus – all of Orbivirus family (*Reoviridae* tribe), Nelson Bay virus, Pulau virus, Broome viruses of Orthoreovirus family (*Reoviridae* tribe) and finally Aqua Preta virus or Parixa virus of *Herpesviridiae* tribe. Some viruses are contagious for humans and are regarded as high-risk agents, e.g. Lyssa virus group, Nipah and Hendra viruses and viral hemorrhagic fever Ebola and Marburg [8, 9, 10].

Chiroptera species are recently associated with *Pasteurella*, *Salmonella*, *Escherichia* and *Yersinia* spp. strains in terms of pathogenic bacterial potential. Bats are capable to induce other bacterial (leptospirosis, salmonellosis) or mycotic infections (histoplasmosis) [11, 12]. There is a limited knowledge on immune system in bats. It is speculated that bats command specific viral inhibitors preventing disease acquire and serving as suitable natural reservoir [13]. Transmission is accomplished by bite, scratching, by saliva, by aerosol containing blood and urine particles but bat dung or *guano* can also be dangerous. Guano could contaminate soil by spores. In equatorial Africa, human consumption of bushmeat including bats has been linked to animal-to-human transmission of such diseases [14, 15, 16].

The majority of all bats are living in colonies in hollows, crevices, foliage, in caves, cavities and even human-made structures or in old estates. Speleologists, divers and other professions should avoid direct and indirect contact with whether hanging or hibernated animals or with excrements. It is recommended not to enter caves, to check stone surfaces and even bush and trees close to caves. Places for camping in nature should also be checked. Regular use of mosquito net protecting against bats too is advisable. Children should be informed not to touch living or dead animals. At sites of infected animals occurrence net devices should be applied to chimney and windows [17, 18].

On the other side one must mention performing vital ecological roles of *pollinating flowers* and dispersing fruit seeds due to bats. Many tropical plant species depend entirely on bats for the distribution of their seeds. Bats are economically important, as they consume insect pests, reducing the need for pesticides. Guano is useful for fertilization or for soap production. Understanding of the echolocation system enabled sonar development.

Viral or Bacterial Diseases Spread Worldwide

Lyssa Viruses

Beside dogs, foxes, raccoons and skunks, bats are frequent animal transmitters of lyssa viruses responsible for rabies occurring worldwide, i.e. fatal human disease [19, 20].

In the United States one to two cases of by bat transmitted rabies in humans are reported yearly. Between 1997 – 2006, nineteen natural infections were reported, 17 attributed to bats. Four patients found bats close to them in their bedrooms, one patient was woken up by an attacking and biting bat, one individual was attacked when leaving home. Three subjects were trying to trap bats incompetently at their home. On the contrary one man took sick animal home to help him. Three other persons in the age of 20, 29 and 64 years died of rabies associated with bats. Death cases due to ignorance are not so rare. Four weeks after onset of diseases the nanny associated it with finding of a bat on floor of children´s room, unfortunately too late and the baby died. Similarly, ten years old child died of rabies in uninstructed family when carrying dead bat out of parent´s bedroom. Particularly in the United States it is very important to inform public on possible transmission of rabies from bat to humans. People have generally positive relation to bats – it is a sign of favorite holiday Halloween – and they are not aware of possible fatal outcomes of contacts with sick animals in principle [21, 22].

The WHO is regularly highlighting not to undervalue the role of bats in rabies epidemic in Europe. Only recently, 32 cases associated with bat transmission were reported – 5 cases in France, 10 in Germany, 3 in Poland, 1 in Spain, 11 in Netherland and 2 in the UK [23].

Not even imported cases of rabies are not so rare. Thirty-four years old Dutch lady acquired rabies and died on day 23 while spending two weeks in Kenya and visiting popular caves with bat colony where she experienced two bleeding scratches [24].

Not treated rabies is fatal in 100% of cases. Vaccination is the only possible diseases prophylaxis.

There are several lyssa viruses in Africa and in India, primarily associated with bats, where current vaccines are not potent [22, 23, 40].

Coronaviruses

Coronarovirus representatives are present in more bat types. These viruses are responsible for mild to moderate cases but also for SARS epidemic in Southeast Asia. The Chinese identified recently viruses in three bat types *Rhinolophus* and which were similar to human SARS CoV. Transmission by saliva or by bite has been supposed. Case of transmission by food intake of food previously present in bat chop was also described. SARS with high morbidity and mortality rates is regarded as a disorder of 21st century. Pandemic spreading from Hong Kong and China has been reported during the first five months of 2003. More than 8 000 people were affected by SARS and 812 of patients died. First in the beginning of summer 2003 pandemic go thunder control due to outstanding efforts of the WHO, the CDC and other national health authorities. Coronaroviruses belong to *Coronaviridae family,* tribe *Coronavirus.* Based on cross serologic reactivity and according to sequential genome analysis *Coronaroviruses* family is divided into three groups. First group produces gastroenteritis and respiratory tract involvement in dogs, cats and in swines. Human coronarovirus 229E is included in this group. Second group represents viruses responsible for diseases in cattle, mouse hepatitis. Human coronarovirus OC43 is also representative of this group. Finally bird viruses create third group (infectious bronchitis in birds and other). Following short incubation period (2-7 days) coronaroviruses induce severe gastrointestinal and respiratory tract involvement, affecting liver and nervous system too. Roughly the same incubation period was recorded in SARS. Generally, coronaviruses are highly species specific. In immunocompetent host they are responsible for neutralizing antibodies production and for cell-mediated immune response resulting in infected cells death. Some animal coronaroviruses induce severe systemic diseases (infectious peritonitis in cats, encephalomyelitis in swine, atc.). Viral replication occurs in liver, kidney, lung, spleen, CNS and *medulla oblongata*. Bird and poultry coronaroviruses of the third group are responsible for significant economic losses in poultry breeder [25, 26].

Histoplasmosis

As in previous diseases, worldwide occurrence is also typical for histoplasmosis caused by fungi *Histoplasma capsulatum*. It is typically distributed in areas of birds, dogs, cats, calves, horses, rats and bat excrements. Under such conditions people should wear face masks and use gloves in contacts with animals. Histoplasmosis is defined as lung infection, spreaded by aerosol inhalation containing microspores of *H. capsulatum*. Clinical presentation is similar to pneumonia. However, asymptomatic course is frequently present. In immunocompromised patients it could be dangerous to neglect management and follow-up [27, 28, 29, 30].

Leptospirosis

In 2008 the European Union reported totally 608 cases of leptospirosis (bacterial infection). Five hundred and ninety-nine cases inclusively were confirmed by lab methods and reported in 26 countries of the European Union. Such data present 0.15 cases per 100.000 inhabitants. It is typically a seasonal disease occurring between July and October and affecting all age groups (highest incidence in the 45-64 age group). Most cases were identified in Germany, Romania, Poland and Slovenia. Main source of disease are rodents, calves and bats (urine). Such infection is only rarely fatal for humans. It is usually seen in farmers and in vets or at slaughters. Gloves and protective measures for eyes, nose and mouth are necessary [3, 22, 23].

Salmonelosis

The salmonella infection is again a worldwide topic. The diseases is induced by intake of contaminated food, transmission from person to person, by contaminated water and due to exposition in environment or to animals are described. Frequently it is attributed to reptiles and cold-blooded, particularly to different exotic representatives. In the US 1.4 million cases are reported annually, in this number 74 000 cases are attributed to reptiles and amphibians. There are no such specific data available in Europe but generally approximately 150.000 cases per year are indicated. In 2008 year, 103 cases per 100.000 inhabitants were reported in the Czech Republic. *Pteropus* family was identified as potential source of *Salmonella enterica*, Typhi serotype in Bangladesh. Infection of bats is mainly attributed to contaminated water [3].

Locally Distributed Diseases

Viral Hemorrhagic Fever Ebola and Marburg

In contrast to worldwide distributed diseases mentioned above, filoviruses inducing viral hemorrhagic fever Ebola and Marburg are located specifically (Africa, Asia). Host was unknown for many years. According to recent knowledge fruit bats are regarded as reservoir and transmission vector of major part of filoviruses in Africa [31, 32]. Sequences of Zaire Ebola strain (ZEBOV) were frequently identified in fruit bats - *Hypsignathus monstrosus, Epomops franqueti* and *Myonycteris torquata*. Sequence of Marburg virus were also identified in frugivorous bats - *Rousettus aegyptiacus* and in insectivorous bats - *Rhinolophus eloquens* a *Miniopterus inflatus.* These animals infected by natural way or experimentally infected by Ebola and Marburg viruses are characterized by an asymptomatic course (in contrast to primates and humans) but excrete virus for 3 weeks. Unforeseen epidemics time after time mainly in countries as Congo, Sudan, Gabon, Republic of South Africa, Ivory Coast, Uganda, Philippines take its course. They are often associated with male involvement – mining workers. Specific culture habits and rituals of existing communities facilitate spreading of lethal infection (e.g. decedent ablutions before funeral). The typical case is a recent Ebola epidemic (close to ZEBOV strain in sequence) in Guinea, Liberia and Sierra Leone. Specific problem in west Africa associated with infection combat is, beside high migration rate, favourite bat and fruit bat consummation in dried form or special sharp pepper soup served with local distilled beverage (gourmet delicacy) [33, 34, 35]. Several thousand infection cases were reported since virus discovery where more than 2/3 of cases died.

Africa is not the only continent for occurrence of high risk viruses. Recently 267 bats *Rousettus leschenaultii* from cave system in Asian Bangladesh were tested – blood, saliva, urine and excrement specimens were positive for antibodies in five animals. Virus isolation was not successful, so it was not possible to analyze genome sequence and compare it (the same strain or a new variant).

Imported infections are described out of Africa - in the 2008 Dutch tourist died of Marburg virus imported from Uganda. There was a similar course in an American tourist visiting Uganda too. Both individuals visited by fruit bats colonized caves.

The new Ebola-like filovirus was described in bat tissue specimen of *Miniopterus schreibersii* (dead animals from Cueva del Llovia caves in Spain) by American and Spanish scientists. The isolated filovirus, Lloviu virus (LLOV) was called according to finding place as Cueva del Lloviu – Cuevavirus. The Cuevavirus is different genetically from other Marburg and Ebola viruses and it is the first filovirus in Europe not imported from endemic area of Africa [32].

The NIAID (National Institute of Allergy and Infectious Diseases) develops Ebola vaccine on base of attenuated virus of vesicular stomatitis containing sequential part of specific protein of Ebola genome. It is a recombinant vector vaccine where viral vector stimulates immune system of immunized. Test with experimental vaccine proved stimulating effects in primates. However difficulties in handling with virus under the highest protection regimen (BSL-4, Biosafety Level) significantly complicate and decelerate research progress.

Nipah and Hendra Viruses

The Nipah and Hendra viruses, included in the same virus family *Paramyxoviridae* and the same tribe *Henipavirus,* present other specific problem. Nipah virus is a causative agent for viral encephalitis, isolated for the first time in 1988 during encephalitis and respiratory tract epidemic in Malaysia (village Sungai Nipah) and in Singapore. Spread of disease occurred in population with close contact with swine (swine farm workers). In 1999 Malaysia affected by significant Nipah epidemic when it was necessary to kill more than 1 million of pigs. Three hundred individuals suffered from disease and 100 of them died. Economic impact of this epidemic was immense. In 2001 Nipah virus occurred in Bangladesh and India. In India, the very first nosocomial transmission route was confirmed. It seems recently that many cases of infection (including fatal ones) are associated with toddy consumption. It is collected to unprotected container on palm trees and fruit bats sip it at night while contaminating product [36].

Hendra virus (family *Paramyxoviridae*, tribe *Henipavirus)* is responsible for viral hendra diseases of respiratory tract and for diseases with neurological involvement. The virus was isolated for the first time in 1994 from clinical specimen collected during epidemic infection in humans and horses in Hendra district in Australian Brisbane. Fruit bats of *Pteropus* genus present a natural reservoir. Horses are affected by food contaminated by urine, saliva or biological products released during bat delivery (transmission by excrements has not been proved yet). Humans are affected by close contacts with body fluids of horse. Next, still sporadic way of transmission, was described in infected horse and dog. Transmission from dog to human has not been reported yet [37, 38].

Flu Viruses

According to CDC study finding of flu viruses presents local problem in Latin and South America. In this study bats of *Artibeus planirostris* kind were detected as reservoir of H17N10 and H18N11 flu viruses in Peru. Positive results of rectal swab specimen were found examining 114 captured animals. A similar finding concerning H17N10 strain was published in Guatemala. It seems that bat population in Latin and South America serves as flu viruses reservoir of different genetic diversity and it is definitely sure to continue in such study types [2, 39].

Hepatotropic Viruses

Hepatotropic viruses were present in isolated and sequenced serum and liver biopsy specimen of together 3,080 bats (*Uroderma bilobatum, Hipposideros of Ruber, Rhinolophus alcyone*) from Panama, Brasilia, Gabon, Ghana, Germany, Papua-New Guinea and from Australia [2].

Conclusion

Numbers of publications and trials analyzing *Chiroptera* order as reservoir and transmitter of microbiological agents as well as "spill over" topic (including transmission of infection from Asian to European endemic *Chiroptera* order representatives) have been increased. Similarly discussion on bats as human food source or specific bats utilization in China´s traditional medicine and possible association with high infectious risk in humans. Migration of these mammalian together with global traveling can change point of view of individual countries in different continents, including Europe in a easy way. No doubt that common availability of intercontinental travelling, migration of population, accelerated transit of large human individuals as a results of expanding air traffic opened new possibilities for viral diseases spreading to other geographical distribution.

As reflected in this article, there are possible transmission risks of viral and bacterial infections from infected animal of *Chiroptera* order to humans following contact. It is necessary to respect safety measures, to limit manipulation and direct contact with animals, to avoid possible animal bites and in given cases to appeal professionals and to disposal activities to them.

References

[1] Horacek I. Flying mammals. *Academia;* Prague, Czech Republic, 1985.

[2] Wong S, Lau S, Woo P, Yuen KY. Bats as a continuing source of emerging infections in humans. *Rev Med Virol,* 2007; 17: 67-91.

[3] Amengual B, Bourhy H, Lopez-Roig M, Serra-Cobo J. Temporal dynamics of European bat Lyssavirus type I and survival of Myotis myotis bats in natural colonies. *Plos One*, 2007; 2: e566.

[4] Shankar V R, Bowen A, Davis A D, Rupprecht C E, OShea T J. Rabies in a captive colony of big brown bats. J *Wild Dis*, 2004; 40: 403-413.

[5] Cryan P M. Seasonal distribution of migratory tree bats in North America. *J Mammal*, 2003; 84: 579-593.

[6] Kunz T H, Parsons S. Ecological and behavioural methods for the study of bats. *John Hopkins University Press, Baltimore,* 2009; 6: 476-488.

[7] Luis A D, Hudson P J. Hibernation patterns in mammals: a role for bacterial growth? *Funct Ecol,* 2006; 20: 471-477.

[8] Daszak P, Cunningham A A, Hyatt AD. Emerging infectious diseases of wildlife. *Science*, 2000; 287: 443-449.

[9] Hayman D T.S. Ecology of zoonotic infectious diseases in bats. *Blackwell Verlag GmbH,* 2013; 60: 2-21.

[10] Drexler J.F, Corman V M, Wegner T, Tateno A F, Zerbinati R M, Gloza Rausch F, Seebens A, Muller M A, Drosten C. Amplification of emerging viruses in a bat colony. *Emerg Infect Dis,* 2011; 17: 449-456.

[11] Duke-Sylvestr S M, Bolzoni L, Real L A. Stong seasonality produces spatial asynchrony in the outbreak of infectious diseases. *J. R. Soc. Interface*, 2011; 8: 817-825.

[12] Breed A C, Field H E, Smith C S, Edmonston J, Meers J. Bats without borders; long distance movements and implications for disease risk managment. *Ecohealth*, 2010; 7: 204-212.

[13] http://www.cdc.gov/features/bats/

[14] 14.Childs J E. Zoonotic viruses of wildlife. *Arch Virol Suppl*, 2004; 3: 1-11.

[15] NaharN.R, Sultana E S, Gurley M J, Hossain J, Luby S.P. Date palm sap collection. *Ecohealth,* 2011; 7: 196-203.

[16] Lloyd Smith J O, Schreiber,S J, Kopp P E, Getz W M. Superspreading and the effect of individual variation on disease emergence. *Nature*, 2005; 438: 355-359.

[17] Boots M, Hudson P J, Sasaki A. Large shift in pathogen virulence relate to host population structure. *Science,* 2004; 303: 842-844.

[18] Muller T, Cox J, Peter,W, Schafer R, Johnson,N, McElhinney L M, Geue J L, Tjørnehøj, K, Fooks A R. Spill-over of European bat lyssavirus type 1 into a stone marten (Martes foina) in Germany. *J Vet Med B Infect Dis Vet Pub Healt,* 2004; 51: 49-54.

[19] Mondul A M, Krebs J W, Childs J E. Trends in national surveillance for rabies among bats in the United States. *J Am Vet Med Assoc,* 2003; 222: 633-639.

[20] Lloyd-Smith J.O, George D, Pepin K M, Pitzer V E, Pulliam J.R, Dobson A P, Hudson P J, Grenfell B T. Epidemic dynamics at the human animal interface. *Science*, 2009; 326: 1362-1367.

[21] Hamspon K, Dushoff J, Cleaveland S, Haydon D T, Kaare M, Parker C, Dobson A. Transmission dynamics and prospects for the elimination of canine rabies. *Plos Biol*, 2009; 7: e1000053.

[22] 22.http://www.cdc.gov/rabies/bats/index.html

[23] 23.http://www.who.int/rabies/resources/Executive_Summary_Rabies_Consultation_Final.pdf?ua=1

[24] Fooks A R, McElhinney L M, Pounder D J, Finnegan C.J, Mansfield K, Johnson N, Brookes S M, Parsons G, White K, McIntyre P G, Nathwani D. Case report: isolation of a European bat lyssavirus type 2a from a fatal human case of rabies encephalitis. *J Med Virol,* 2003; 71: 281-289.

[25] Li W, Shi Z, Yu M, Ren W, Smith C, Epstein J H, Wang H, Crameri G, Hu Z, Zhan H, Zhang., McEachern J, Field H, Daszak P, Eaton B T, Zhang S, Wang L F. Bats are natural reservoirs of SARS-like coronaviruses. *Science,* 2005; 310: 676-679.

[26] Osborne C. P, Cryan M, OShea T J, Oko L M, Ndaluka C, Calisher C H, Berlung A D, Klavetter M L, Bowen R A, Holmes K V, Dominguez S R.. Alphacoronaviruses in New World bats, prevalence, persistence, phylogeny and potential for interaction with humans. *PLoS One*, 2011; 6: e19156.

[27] Anderson R M, May R M. Population biology of infectious diseases. *Nature*, 1979; 280: 361-367

[28] Hayman D T S. Ecology of zoonotic infectious diseases in bats. *Zoonoses and Public Health*, 2013; 60: 2-21.

[29] Wu D, Tu, C, Xin C, Xuan H, Meng Q, Liu Y, Yu Y, Guan Y, Jiang Y, Yin X, Crameri G, Wang M, Li C, Liu S, Liao M, Feng L, Xjang H, Sun J, Chen J, Sun Y, Gu S, Liu N, Fu D, Eaton B T, Wang L F, Kong, X. Civets are equally susceptible to experimental infection by two different severe acute respiratory syndrome coronavirus isolates. *J Virol*, 2005; 79: 2620-2625.

[30] Tu C, Crameri G, Kong X, Chen J, Sun Y, Yu M, Xiang H, Xia X, Liu S, Ren T, Yu Y, Eaton B T, Xuan H, Wang L F. Antibodies to SARS coronavirus in civets. *Emerg Infect Dis,* 2004; 10: 2244-2248.

[31] Špliňo M, Boštíková V. Přenos Ebola viru aerosolem z prasat na primáty. *Vakcinologie*, 2013; 2: 83-84.

[32] Špliňo, M., Boštíková, V. Objev Ebola-like viru u netopýrů ve Španělsku. Vakcinologie, 2012; 2: 80-81.

[33] Pourrut X, Kumulungui B, Wittmann T, Moussavou G, Delicat A, Yaba P. The natural history of Ebola virus in Africa. *Microbes Infect*; 2005; 7: 1005-1014.

[34] Peterson,A T, Carroll DS, Mills J N, Johnson K M. Potenital mammalian filovirus reservoirs. *Emerg Infect Dis*, 2004;10: 2073-2081.

[35] Keeling M, Rohani P. Modeling Infectious Diseases in humans and animals. *Princeton University Press*, 2008.

[36] Hsu.P, Hossain M J, Parashar D, Ali M, Ksiazek T G, Kuzmin I, Niezgoda M, Rupprecht, C, Bresee J, Breiman R F Nipah virus encephalitis reemergence, Bangladesh. *Emerg Infect. Dis*, 2004; 10: 2082-2087.

[37] Halpin K, Young P L, Field H E, Mackenzie J S. Isolation of Hendra virus from pteropis bats. *J GenVirol*, 2000; 81: 1927-1932.

[38] Halpin K, Hyatt A D, Fogarty D, Middleton D, Bingham J H, Epstein S, Rahman A, Hughes T, Smith C, Field H E, Daszak P. Pteropid bats are confirmed as the reservoir hosts of henipaviruses: a comprehensive experimental study of virus transmission. *Am J Trop Med Hyg,* 2011; 85: 946-951.

[39] Tong S, Zhu X, Li Y, Shi M, Zhang J, Bourgeois M. New World bats harbor diverse influenza A viruses. *PLoS Patho*, 2013; 9: e1003657.

[40] www.cdc.gov/mmwr/preview/mmwrhtml/rr5703a1.htm (human rabies prevention)

In: Hemorrhagic Fever
Editor: Shirley R. Edwards

ISBN: 978-1-63482-791-1

Chapter IV

South American Arenaviral Hemorrhagic Fevers

B. I. Stephan, A. F. De Ganzó, M. E. Lozano and S. E. Goñi*

[1]Área de Virosis Emergentes y Zoonóticas (AVEZ), Laboratorio de Ingeniería Genética y Biología Celular y Molecular (LIGBCM), Instituto de Microbiología Básica y Aplicada (IMBA), Dto. Ciencia y Tecnología, Universidad Nacional de Quilmes, Buenos Aires, Argentina

Abstract

The New World clade of the *Arenaviridae* family includes several hemorrhagic fever viruses which are important emerging pathogens in South America. The four most significant members of the viral family in this aspect are Junín virus (JUNV), causative agent of the Argentine Hemorrhagic Fever (AHF); Machupo virus (MACV), etiological agent of Bolivian Hemorrhagic Fever (BHF); Guanarito virus (GTOV), which causes Venezuelan Hemorrhagic Fever (VeHF) and Sabiá virus (SABV), causing Brazilian Hemorrhagic Fever (BrHF). Although they are currently constrained to relatively small geographic regions, the global concern regarding these infections is in rise since the outbreak of the Ebola epidemic. Here we describe the clinical symptoms of these viral

* Corresponding Author. Email: sandra.goni@unq.edu.ar.

diseases and the most widely used diagnostic methods for the correct identification of the pathogen involved. The analysis of recent epidemiological data in conjunction with climatic and cultural changes shows the imprint of human activity on the environment and can easily be related to the viral emergence.

Introduction

Viral Hemorrhagic Fevers in the Americas

The recent outbreaks of viral infectious disease, particularly the Ebola epidemic in Africa, have focused the attention on other emerging viruses worldwide. Among those of greatest harm potential are the causative agents of the Viral Hemorrhagic Fevers (VHFs). VHF refers to a collection of infectious diseases that affect humans, resulting in very similar symptoms. Regardless of the virus involved the disease progresses to a severe multisystem syndrome, principally with fever and bleeding risk.

The know VHF viruses are members of only five out of the over 100 existing viral families: arenaviruses (JUNV, MACV, GTOV, SABV and Lassa virus), bunyaviruses (Crimean-Congo virus), filoviruses (Marburg and Ebola viruses), flaviviruses (Yellow Fever and Dengue viruses) and paramyxoviruses (Hendra and Nipah viruses) [1]. They all have an RNA genome and a lipid envelope, as well as a dependence on a non-human natural reservoir. This last feature translates into a geographic restriction to areas populated by the host [2]. Also, since humans are not the natural reservoir, they usually become infected via contact with a virus-carrying host. In consequence, outbreaks among the human population are sporadic and hard to predict.

In South America only the flaviviruses and arenaviruses (with the exception of Lassa, present mainly in Africa) cause VHFs. The Dengue virus had been restricted to isolated areas in the Caribbean Islands, as a result of mosquito elimination campaigns of the Pan American Health Organization (PAHO) during the 1950s and 1960s. However, the absence of similar policies in Africa and Asia together with a relaxation of the control measures in the Americas and the adaptation of the mosquito to the urban environ allowed the reintroduction of the virus in this area [3]. In consequence, in the last decades the number of cases of Dengue Fever (DF) has increased dramatically. There is no effective treatment against the viral multiplication and the main concern is to alleviate the symptoms in order to avoid complications and secondary infections. Several vaccines are being developed, but so far they are in different clinical trial stages [4].

The other VHF caused by a flavivirus in South America is Yellow Fever (YF). This virus is transmitted to the humans by the same mosquito as the Dengue virus. Therefore, during the years of the PAHO campaign, this disease was also severely reduced [5]. However, the existence of a so-called sylvan cycle, which involves monkeys and forest mosquitos, still remained as an alternative source of infection [6]. The reintroduction of the DF mosquito did not pose such a great risk of YF outbreaks because there is an effective vaccine in use [7]. The fact that it is a cheap vaccine permitted the massive inoculation of risk populations in all of South America. However, after several years without outbreaks a number of factors combined to produce the increase of cases [8]. As with DF, there is no specific treatment for YF and patient care is based on symptom mitigation.

Infections with LASV or the VHF causing filoviruses and bunyaviruses occasionally appear in South America, but only as imported cases. The main areas affected by the other VHF viruses are different regions of the Old World where the non-human reservoirs are found.

In this chapter we review the South American Arenaviral Hemorrhagic Fevers (SAHFs) and the importance of recent changes in human activities on their epidemiology.

The Arenavirus family is composed of two great clusters, based on serological, molecular and geographical criteria: the Old World and the New World group [9]. The latter is divided into four different clades (A, B, C and A/rec) with several members in each of them. All of the SAHF causing viruses are members of the clade B, along with other arenaviruses that so far have not been reported as human pathogens [10]. They all have a very small endemic area because of a conjunction of factors (Figure 1). First, arenaviruses have a narrow host range, infecting a few or even just one rodent species [11]. Second, the number of infected rodents is usually low and they are not widespread on the American continent. Last, the human being is a dead-end host of the virus and acquires the infection almost exclusively through close contact with the rodents or their excretions. Taken together, these characteristics account for the reduced regions of endemicity of most arenaviruses. The one exception is the Lymphocytic Choriomeningitis Virus, which has *Mus musculus* as a reservoir and can be found everywhere around the globe.

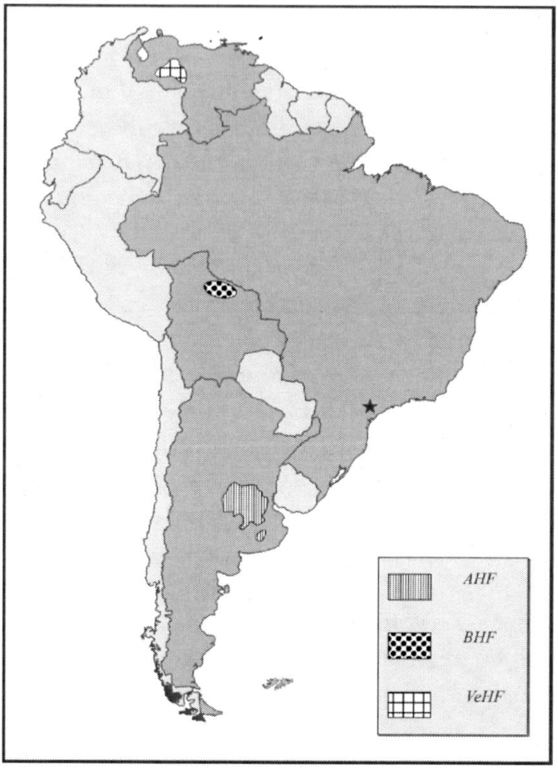

Figure 1. Endemic regions of the SAHFs. The map shows the different regions of South America where the outbreaks of hemorrhagic fevers have occurred. The star in Brazil represents the city of São Paulo, where the only case of non-laboratory related BrHF was reported.

Molecular and Cell Biology of Arenaviruses

The particles of the arenaviruses are spherical in shape, with an approximate diameter of 120 nm [12]. The outer layer is a lipid membrane with spike-like projections that are the viral glycoproteins. In a cross-section these virions have a grainy aspect due to the high number of ribosomes included from the host cell [13]. This sandy characteristic is the origin of the viral family name (from the Latin, "arena" means "sand"). The genomic material comprises two single-stranded RNA segments of different sizes. The large (L) segment has approx. 7200 nucleotides while the small (S) segment has close to 3600 nucleotides [14]. Both share the same basic organization of coding and non-coding regions, with two open reading frames in opposite orientations [15] separated by an intergenic region and flanked by the non-coding ends (5' and 3' untranslated regions). The L segment codes for the viral replicase (L protein) on the 3' side and the matrix protein (Z) on the 5' side. The S segment encodes the precursor of the glycoproteins (GPC, 5') and the nucleoprotein (N, 3'). These RNAs have a great tendency to form highly complex secondary structures through hybridization of regions within the same strand and are usually associated with the viral protein N [16].

All the viral proteins are included in the virion and have multiple functions [16–18]. The genomic segments associate with many molecules of the N protein to form the ribonucleoproteins (RNPs). These RNPs, together with a small number of L proteins and numerous cellular components, are covered by a coat of matrix protein. Beyond this there is a lipidic layer derived from the cellular membrane which includes the viral glycoproteins [20].

Clinical Disease

Humans can acquire a SAHF virus through contact with infected rodent excretions (urine or saliva) by inhalation of aerosolized particles or ingestion of contaminated food. Within the body, the clade B arenaviruses require the cellular surface protein TfRI as a specific receptor for cell entry [21]. This protein is involved in iron uptake and is present in a wide range of cell types. It is expressed at a high level on very active or dividing cells (including those of the immune system) as well as on endothelia [22]. The tropism of the SAHF viruses can partly be explained by the greater availability of the receptor on these cell types. Principal targets for the infection are macrophages and several cells of the lymphatic system, allowing for a rapid spread inside the infected organism [23]. The infection of endothelial cells leads to dysfunctions without apparent cytopathic effect [24].

The initial multiplication of the virus generally occurs in the lungs, from where it disseminates to the lymphatic system [25]. These replication rounds don't leave significant tissue damage and are asymptomatic. The arenaviruses have an incubation period of 7 to 14 days, depending on species and host status. Thereafter begins the SAHF proper, with unspecific clinical manifestations (asthenia, mucosal and skin rashes, dizziness, fever, muscular pain and lymph node swelling) [26]. At this stage it is very hard to have a correct diagnosis since the pathogen identification depends on very specific molecular methods. One week to ten days after onset of the SAHF the patient worsens, with renal, gastrointestinal, cardiovascular and neurologic involvement. In summary, the most frequent and characteristic manifestations of the SAHF are fever and hypotension with occasional hemorrhages, platelet dysfunction, lymphopenia, thrombocytopenia and hepatic but not vascular damage. The virus infects macrophages and dendritic cells, generating elevated levels of cytokines and interferons [27].

The elimination of the virus depends mainly on the humoral immune response, through neutralizing antibodies [28]. If the patient is unable to clear the infection, the disease progresses to a hemorrhagic shock syndrome that is fatal in up to 30% of the cases.

The pathological lesions are principally multiple hemorrhages in subcutaneous tissue, gastrointestinal mucosa and various organs (liver, lung and kidney among others). There are no apparent pathologies to the central nervous system in spite of the neurologic manifestations that frequently occur [29]–[32]. The involvement of lymphatic cells can often derive in secondary bacterial infections. This complicates diagnosis and can mask the specific symptoms of the SAHF [33].

The characteristic hemorrhagic syndrome that ensues in severe cases is not completely understood. It is attributed to alterations in the coagulation and an important thrombocytopenia, in conjunction with damage to the vascular tissue, induced by cytokines and the viral multiplication. As a difference with other viral hemorrhagic fevers, there is usually no disseminated intravascular coagulation [34]. In fatal cases, besides the typical hemorrhagic syndrome elements described above, there are low activity levels of platelets. Evidence of the existence of an inhibitor of platelet aggregation has been found in the plasma of infected patients, but its precise nature is still to be determined [35]. Another distinctive feature of fatal cases is immunosuppression due to viral activity.

The suppression is caused by complex mechanisms that involve several factors, including the early infection of dendritic cells. Some fatal patients do not develop the hemorrhagic syndrome and have mainly neurological symptoms. However, the molecular and pathological bases for the clinical manifestations of the nervous system are largely unknown [36].

The patients that recover from a SAHF usually have an antiviral immune response by the second week after onset of the disease. The convalescent plasma contains elevated titers of neutralizing antiviral IgGs [37]. In most cases there are no lasting effects of the infection upon recovery, even in patients that had neurologic syndrome.

Diagnosis

The similarity in the clinical manifestations of the majority of the viral hemorrhagic fevers makes it practically impossible to arrive at a positive diagnosis without specific laboratory tests. Traditionally, the most accepted method for identification is the viral isolation through cultivation *in vitro*. However this technique is labor-intensive and requires specialized equipment, highly trained personnel as well as tissue or fluid samples containing viable virions. The samples must be harvested in the precise window when virus shedding is happening and stored in appropriate conditions to ensure the survival of the viruses.

There are two types of methods most commonly used with these viruses: immunoaffinity based and polymerase chain reaction (PCR) based. As these pathogens have RNA genomes, the first stage has to be a reverse transcription (RT). The advances in PCR reagents have allowed for a one-step approach which makes it possible to convert the RNA template in DNA and amplify the specific target region in the same tube, without having to open it. The sample preparation has been adapted to permit the use of whole blood without complex processing or high risk for the laboratory workers [38]. More recently, several real time PCRs have been developed that have the benefit of being more sensitive and allowing quantitative results [39], [40]. The greatest advantage of this type of technique is that it can be used to establish an early diagnosis, since a low number of viral genomes are sufficient to arrive at a positive conclusion. Other closely related methods use specific hybridization of oligonucleotides in a microarray format that permits testing for a very large number of pathogens simultaneously [41].

The serological methods include several different types of assays for the detection of viral antigens or antibodies against the viral agent. The majority of these can employ either wild type virus or recombinant proteins. The enzyme-linked immunosorbent assay (ELISA) format is applicable for the detection of IgG or IgM in the patients' fluids if the whole viral particle or a suitable viral component is immobilized on the plaque. The other method is the indirect immunofluorescence assay (IFA) which utilizes fixed, virus infected cells to bind the specific antibodies [42]. In order to avoid the risk of pathogen manipulation the more recent assays use cells expressing highly immunogenic, recombinant viral proteins. The images obtained with an IFA show a signal pattern that is characteristic of each virus, but the correct interpretation of the results requires a trained eye.

Another ELISA type test is used for detection of viral antigens employing polyclonal or monoclonal antibodies (singly or in combination). The captured antigen can be the whole viral particle or any of its components, proteins as well as genomes. The possibility of producing even small fragments of the viral proteins as recombinant polypeptides and raising monoclonal or polyclonal antibodies against them gives a practically unlimited versatility to this technique. With the correct design it can allow the differentiation of closely related pathogens or the simultaneous probing for a high number of microorganisms [43], [44].

The last type of assay, traditionally used as a golden standard for a great number of viruses, is the neutralization test. This method uses the antibodies in a patients' sample to bind the viral surface antigens and so "neutralize" the infective potential of that particle. The presence of neutralizing immunoglobulins is indicative of protection against a new infection with the same pathogen and is a very valuable criterion for the efficacy of a vaccine. These assays are normally performed with wild type virus because the natural infectivity is a key element in the determination [45]. The recombinant alternative are pseudotyped, replication incompetent viruses that bare the same surface antigens as the pathogen of interest [46].

As a general rule, the tests that identify viral components are more useful for early diagnosis, when viral multiplication is occurring near the entry point and the infection has not spread far. Under those circumstances the application of the treatment options produces very good results. When the infection has progressed and a diagnosis of hemorrhagic fever has been established through the clinical manifestations, the serological assays are employed to determine the particular pathogen involved. Nevertheless, there are cases that do not arrive at a positive identification because some patients fail to seroconvert.

Treatment

Fundamentally, patient care is based on supportive treatment to minimize the consequences of the virus induced damages. However, this is not enough to reduce the high mortality rates (up to 30%) or improve the patients' prognosis. The great number of cases identified during the initial years of the AHF emergence showed the necessity of finding further treatment. During that time (1950s) the administration of convalescent plasma as a means of lessening the severity of the disease was a common practice for cases of other viral infections [47]. Consequently, this therapy was used almost from the beginning based on previous experimental results. When administered near the onset of the symptoms (less than 8 days), this treatment can reduce mortality rates to 1-2% [48]. Unfortunately, there are several drawbacks including a late neurological syndrome that appears in 10% of the cases [49]. Other disadvantages are the difficulty to maintain an adequate stock of plasma and the high risk of transfusion-borne pathogens.

The specific therapies against the SAHFs have only begun to be developed in the last two decades. The greater availability of high throughput screening methods allowed for shorter times and lower costs in that particular research field. The antiviral drug Rivabirin (also known as Virazole), first described for its therapeutic potential in 1972 [50] has been used against the SAHF viruses since the 1980s. Its usefulness was tested for patients outside the timeframe for the existing therapy, i.e. as a prophylaxis in cases of exposure to the virus and for patients with more than 8 days of evolution [51].

Several inhibitors of viral entry or replication have been proposed as viable therapeutic agents [52]–[55]. Also, other types of molecules like antibodies and oligonucleotides are being investigated as alternatives to the classic antivirals [56]–[58].

Vaccines

There are no vaccines for the majority of arenaviruses. The notable exceptions are Lassa virus, which has several vaccines in clinical trial stage and JUNV [59]. The history of the JUNV vaccine started in 1958, the year when the virus was discovered to be the causative agent of AHF. During that outbreak a high virulence strain (named XJ) was isolated from a patient [60]. That strain was serially passaged in rodents in Argentina and then taken to the USAMRIID (United States Army Medical Research Institute of Infectious Diseases) laboratories in USA as part of a covenant between the two countries' governments, the PAHO and the UN [61]. The greater capabilities of these facilities made it possible to produce an attenuated JUNV strain in a shorter time. The actual work was performed by the argentine scientists J. Barrera Oro y J. Maiztegui. The whole process was punctually documented and every intermediate strain was stored for future analysis [62], [63]. The resulting vaccine is based on the attenuated virus Candid#1 [64] (Figure 2). By the year 1984 the clinical trials were underway in Argentina with volunteers from the endemic area [65], [66]. These trials continued until 1988 and in 1991 the vaccine started to be used on individuals belonging to high-risk groups.

Finally, in 2007 the complete production of the vaccine doses was shifted to the National Institute for Human Viral Diseases in Argentina [67]. More recently there have been variations in the epidemiology of JUNV that changed the definition of the high-risk groups [68].

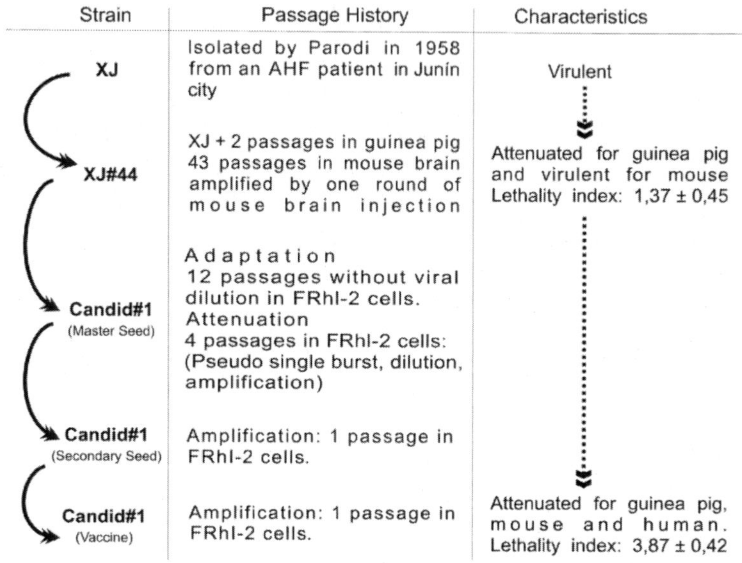

Figure 2. History of the JUNV vaccine. The schematic shows the sequential passages that were made to obtain the final seed, Candid#1.

Epidemiology

Argentine Hemorrhagic Fever (AHF)

The first description of the typical symptoms of AHF was made during an outbreak that took place in the town of Bragado, province of Buenos Aires (Argentina) during the years 1953 to 1955 [69]. However, the isolation of the pathogen responsible was accomplished some time later, in 1956, by two independent research groups [60], [62]. At that moment, the endemic area of AHF occupied only the north of the province of Buenos Aires but rapidly expanded to the north of La Pampa and the south of Santa Fe and Cordoba.

The natural hosts of JUNV are several rodents, principally *Calomys musculinus* and *Calomys laucha*, and in a lesser proportion *Akodon azarae* and *Orizomys flavescens* [70]. The rodents inhabit the principal agricultural region of Argentina, where cereals are cultivated.

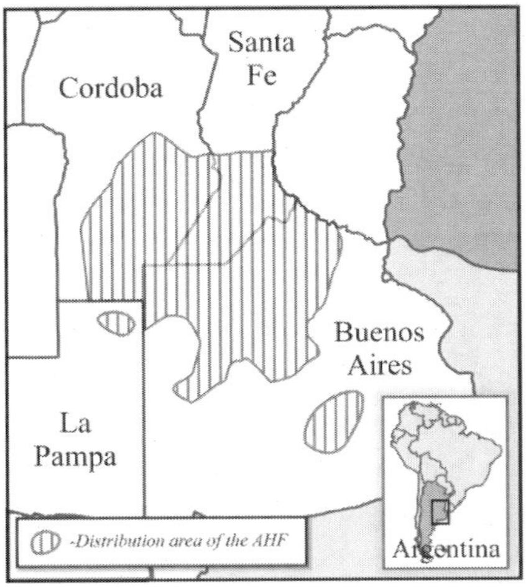

Figure 3. Endemic area of AHF. The map represents part of Argentina, with the region of highest case reports shaded differentially.

The normal conduct of these mice is to keep on the borders of the fields during the stages of plowing and sowing, when the lack of vegetation would leave them exposed. As the crops grow, the rodents move into the fields and stay there until the moment of the harvest. Generally, the gathering of the cereals is done with machinery, which translates into a high mortality for the smaller animals. The surviving individuals flee to the border habitats until a new growth season begins [71]. This cyclic behavior is mirrored in the seasonal incidence of the disease. The greater number of cases occurs during harvest time, when rural workers are closely in contact with the nests and during the successive month, when the rodents are displaced to the border habitats and tend to invade human dwellings [72].

The endemic area of AHF is still expanding (Figure 3), probably due to a multiplicity of factors. First, the area of cultivation of cereals has steadily grown as a result of the high profit possibility of soy crops. This allows the rodents to find adequate living conditions in places they had not established themselves in before. Second, the massive change to a small plant has favored the development of rodents over that of the predatory animals, which are bigger and consequently need larger hiding places to escape from humans. Third, the transportation of crops by truck to the nearest port has brought new persons into the endemic area. The fact that the disease has more than a week of incubation period results in a delay in its onset. The infected individual is probably far from the place of acquisition of the virus by the time the diagnosis is made. Normally this would be considered an imported case, but the steady flow of workers to and from the endemic area has made the situation so frequent that it is treated as an expansion of the AHF region.

The extensive use of the vaccine against JUNV has been highly successful [73]. As a consequence, most of the risk-group population is protected from AHF, leaving little susceptible subjects for the viral infection. In recent years there has been a shift of case numbers, with a higher incidence in women and children [74].

Bolivian Hemorrhagic Fever (BHF)

BHF is a disease found almost exclusively in the district of Beni in Bolivia (Figure 4). The first reported outbreak appeared in 1959 and lasted until 1964. Prior to this there was no testimony of the existence of BHF neither from physicians nor locals [75]. The clinical manifestations clearly pointed to a viral hemorrhagic fever very much like AHF. The causative agent, virus Machupo, was isolated from the spleen of a fatal case in 1963 [76]. That same year an intensive sampling of the local fauna took place in an effort to identify the non-human host. The virus was successfully isolated from only one species: *Calomys callosus* [77]. This rodent inhabits several regions of Bolivia, Brazil, Argentina and Paraguay. However, BHF is endemic to the Beni district and only a handful of cases have been reported elsewhere. An extensive study of *C. callosus* found that the groups that act as reservoirs through the transmission and maintenance of MACV belong to a lineage with independent monophyletic characteristics that differ substantially from the other lineages present in the rest of Bolivia and South America [78].

The great similarity with AHF extends to the form of transmission of the virus from rodents to humans. Also, there are several cases of nosocomial transmission documented, where relatives visiting a BHF patient afterwards developed the disease [79], [80]. In the 1959 outbreak the majority of infected persons were adult males [75]. This was probably related to the way of acquisition of the infection, i. e. the close contact with the rodents' excreta in the fields. In 1963 the outbreak spread from the small villages to the urban center San Joaquín. This was thought to be related with a decrease in the cat population due to DDT poisoning [81]. The smaller number of cats in the urban environ allowed for the establishment of *C. callosus* inside the houses. Having identified the rodents as natural reservoirs, in May-June of 1964 a comprehensive program of rodent control began in the affected area. These measures included not only the capture and extermination with night cages but also the use of poison and traps along with the destruction of nests in every human dwelling.

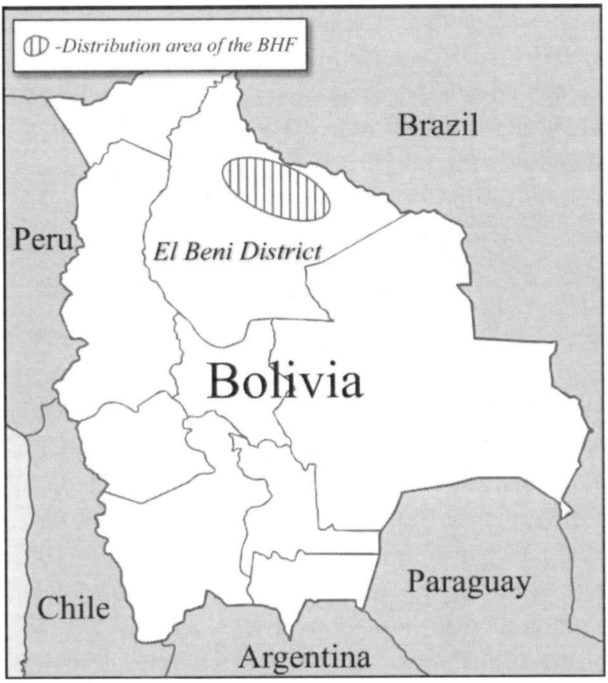

Figure 4. Endemic area of BHF. The map represents the country of Bolivia, with the province of Beni shaded differentially.

The success of the program was seen as soon as two weeks after its initiation, with a marked reduction in case numbers [82]. The importation of cats was another form of rodent population control that contributed to the handling of the BHF outbreak.

In the period of 1965 to 1975 less than 50 cases were reported, testifying to the efficacy of the implemented measures. After this, there came a long period without notified cases, although it is possible that the remoteness of the villages and the scarcity of trained medical attendants converged to under-document sporadic cases. An alarm was raised in 1994 with several isolated cases and one entire family unit with BHF occurring in two month [83]. Luckily this situation did not develop into an outbreak and case reports again quieted down until 2007. Since then, there has been an almost yearly increase in case reports during the month of February and March [84]. This coincides with the end of the rain season, when the lowlands are flooded and rodents flee to the highlands where the cultivated areas are. Also, the expansion of agricultural areas brings more individuals in close contact with the rodents.

In 2004 another arenavirus was isolated from a fatal case derived from a small cluster of BHF near Cochabamba. Although the clinical manifestations were indistinguishable from those caused by the MACV infection, a molecular characterization of the virus permitted the identification of a new species: Chapare virus [85]. It is thought that both BHF viruses coexist in Bolivia, but further studies are required to understand the role of Chapare virus in the diseases' epidemiology.

Brazilian Hemorrhagic Fever (BrHF)

The causative agent of BrHF is the arenavirus Sabiá, with an as yet unidentified host. The virus was first isolated from a fatal case of hemorrhagic fever in an agricultural engineer in São Paulo, in the year 1990 [86]. This isolate was later characterized and one of the technicians involved in the process also developed a severe illness, without fatal outcome [87]. A third case, acquired because of a leak of infectious material in a high speed centrifuge in a biosafety level 3 laboratory, was reported in 1995. The patient was hospitalized, treated with ribavirin and never developed hemorrhagic symptoms [88]. Since then no other cases have been reported, but the manipulation of the virus now requires a biosafety level 4 laboratory. This has hindered further studies with the virus and only few advances have been made since 1996 [89].

VenezuelanHemorrhagic Fever (VeHF)

In September of 1989 an outbreak of a severe hemorrhagic fever began in the state of Portuguesa, municipality of Guanarito, initially thought to be Dengue Fever [90]. However, a re-examination of the etiology discovered a novel arenavirus in the area: GTOV. Prior to this, the cases of VeHF had probably been misdiagnosed due to the presence of hemorrhagic fever flaviviruses in the region.

The central plains of Venezuela are located in the states of Barinas and Portuguesa, and are known as *llanos*. The rural areas of these *llanos* form the endemic region were the human cases of VeHF have been reported (Figure 5). As with other arenaviruses, GTOV has a rodent host responsible for the maintenance of the pathogen in nature. The principal reservoir of GTOV is thought to be the short-tailed cane mouse *Zygodontomys brevicauda* [91], although there is evidence that another rodent species (*Sigmodon alstoni*) plays an important role in the viruses' natural cycle [92]. A study showed a rather high prevalence of antibodies against GTOV in rodents and a low prevalence in humans during the years of that first outbreak [93].

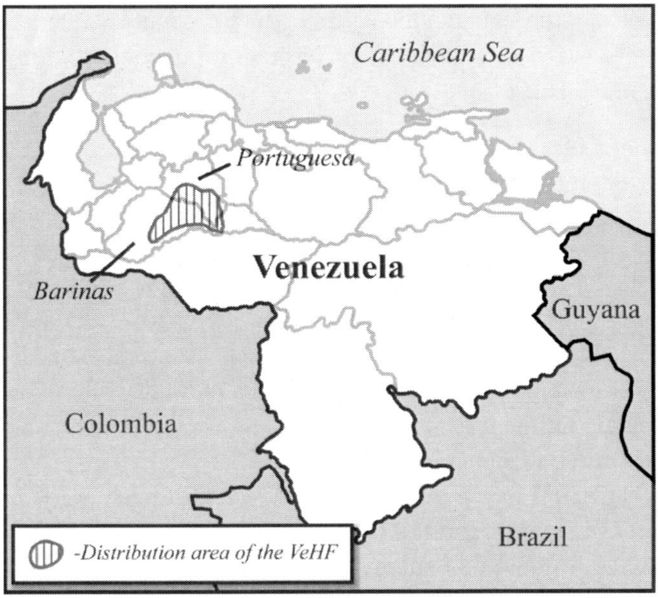

Figure 5. Endemic area of VeHF. The map represents Venezuela, with the region of the llanos in a different shade.

This could be explained by the relatively small opportunities of contact between humans and infected rodents or their excreta. To understand this it is necessary to consider that the municipality of Guanarito has a total surface of more than 2400 km^2 and a population of 24000 people, mostly in rural communities.

The number of VeHF cases reported to the ministry of health between 1989 and 1998 was greater than 200. Over the years, a cyclic pattern emerged, with the majority of cases happening in productive-aged males, at the juncture of the rainy and the dry seasons (November through January) [94]. During that period there is an intense agricultural activity, done mainly by adult males of the local population and imported workers. This suggests that the acquisition of the infection happens away from the family homes. Taking into account that during the last decade of the 20th century a large number of people moved from other areas to the *llanos*, there are several factors that may help to explain the increase of VeHF cases. First, the greater population density made opportunities of human-rodent interactions more frequent. Second, in order to exploit the available land for farming, the existing vegetation (mostly forests) was removed, forcing the rodents into closer contact with the agricultural workers. And thirdly, the abundance of grains and grass favored the sustenance of bigger populations of certain rodents, among them *Z. brevicauda*[95]. All these situations converge to produce a progressive rise in the disease's prevalence.

Conclusion

The SAHF viruses share a great number of characteristics and have very similar dynamics when infecting humans [21], [96]. However, the volume of precise knowledge available for each distinct virus differs substantially. Regardless of the biohazard level, they all have a mortality rate of around 30% when not treated, but there only exists a vaccine for JUNV. The emergence of sporadic cases that are not related in any way to laboratory-acquisition is a proof that the SAHF viruses constitute a latent threat. It is of special importance to fully understand the basis of transmission to be able to establish secure protocols in future epidemics. In 2009 the emergence of an arenavirus produced an outbreak in the south of Africa, with 4 fatal cases out of a total of five [97]. The causative agent was later identified as a novel arenavirus with a high capacity to spread from human to human [98].

The easier access to rapid transportation has permitted massive human migrations in short times, with the consequent alterations in the affected environments. The expansion of urban regions and the deforestation in favor of agricultural activities have wrought changes in the natural habitats of the rodents, bringing them in closer contact with humans. It seems only a matter of time before the occurrence of the next great outbreak of a SAHF. In the meantime, it is very important to learn as much as possible about these viruses to be prepared.

References

[1] "Viral Hemorrhagic Fevers (VHFs)." [Online]. Available: http://www.cdc.gov/vhf/virus-families/index.html.

[2] R. N. Charrel and X. de Lamballerie, "Arenaviruses other than Lassa virus.," *Antiviral Res.*, vol. 57, no. 1–2, pp. 89–100, Jan. 2003.

[3] J. R. Powell and W. J. Tabachnick, "History of domestication and spread of Aedes aegypti - a review.," *Mem. Inst. Oswaldo Cruz*, vol. 108 Suppl, no. August, pp. 11–7, 2013.

[4] R. B. McFee, "Viral hemorrhagic fever viruses.," *Dis. Mon.*, vol. 59, pp. 410–25, 2013.

[5] T. Monath, "Yellow fever and dengue—the interactions of virus, vector and host in the re-emergence of epidemic disease," *Seminars in virology*, vol. 5. pp. 133–145, 1994.

[6] E. De Rodaniche, P. Galindo, and C. M. Johnson, "Isolation of yellow fever virus from Haemagogus lucifer, H. equinus, H.," *Am. J. Trop. Med. Hyg.*, vol. 6, pp. 681–685, 1957.

[7] F. X. Heinz and K. Stiasny, "Flaviviruses and flavivirus vaccines," *Vaccine*, vol. 30, no. 29, pp. 4301–4306, 2012.

[8] C. V. F. Carrington and A. J. Auguste, "Evolutionary and ecological factors underlying the tempo and distribution of yellow fever virus activity," *Infection, Genetics and Evolution*, vol. 13. Elsevier B.V., pp. 198–210, 2013.

[9] R. N. Charrel, X. de Lamballerie, and S. Emonet, "Phylogeny of the genus Arenavirus.," *Curr. Opin. Microbiol.*, vol. 11, no. 4, pp. 362–8, Aug. 2008.

[10] H. Choe, S. Jemielity, J. Abraham, S. R. Radoshitzky, and M. Farzan, "Transferrin receptor 1 in the zoonosis and pathogenesis of New World hemorrhagic fever arenaviruses.," *Curr. Opin. Microbiol.*, vol. 14, no. 4, pp. 476–82, Aug. 2011.

[11] M. D. Bowen, C. J. Peters, and S. T. Nichol, "Phylogenetic analysis of the Arenaviridae: patterns of virus evolution and evidence for cospeciation between arenaviruses and their rodent hosts.," *Mol. Phylogenet. Evol.*, vol. 8, no. 3, pp. 301–16, Dec. 1997.

[12] F. a Murphy, P. a Webb, K. M. Johnson, S. G. Whitfield, and W. a Chappell, "Arenoviruses in Vero cells: ultrastructural studies.," *J. Virol.*, vol. 6, no. 4, pp. 507–18, Oct. 1970.

[13] B. W. Neuman, B. D. Adair, J. W. Burns, R. A. Milligan, M. J. Buchmeier, and M. Yeager, "Complementarity in the supramolecular design of arenaviruses and retroviruses revealed by electron cryomicroscopy and image analysis.," *J. Virol.*, vol. 79, no. 6, pp. 3822–30, Mar. 2005.

[14] P. D. Ghiringhelli, R. V Rivera-Pomar, M. E. Lozano, O. Grau, and V. Romanowski, "Molecular organization of Junin virus S RNA: complete nucleotide sequence, relationship with other members of the Arenaviridae and unusual secondary structures.," *J. Gen. Virol.*, vol. 72 (Pt 9), pp. 2129–41, Sep. 1991.

[15] D. D. Auperin, V. Romanowski, M. Galinski, D. H. L. Bishopt, and D. H. Bishop, "Sequencing studies of pichinde arenavirus S RNA indicate a novel coding strategy, an ambisense viral S RNA.," *J. Virol.*, vol. 52, no. 3, pp. 897–904, Dec. 1984.

[16] P. R. Young and C. R. Howard, "Fine structure analysis of Pichinde virus nucleocapsids.," *J. Gen. Virol.*, vol. 64 (Pt 4), pp. 833–42, Apr. 1983.

[17] S. K. Fehling, F. Lennartz, and T. Strecker, "Multifunctional nature of the arenavirus RING finger protein Z.," *Viruses*, vol. 4, no. 11, pp. 2973–3011, Nov. 2012.

[18] J. M. Levingston Macleod, A. D'Antuono, M. E. Loureiro, J. C. Casabona, G. a Gomez, and N. Lopez, "Identification of two functional domains within the arenavirus nucleoprotein.," *J. Virol.*, vol. 85, no. 5, pp. 2012–23, Mar. 2011.

[19] B. Morin, B. Coutard, M. Lelke, F. Ferron, R. Kerber, S. Jamal, A. Frangeul, C. Baronti, R. Charrel, X. de Lamballerie, C. Vonrhein, J. Lescar, G. Bricogne, S. Günther, and B. Canard, "The N-terminal domain of the arenavirus L protein is an RNA endonuclease essential in mRNA transcription.," *PLoS Pathog.*, vol. 6, no. 9, p. e1001038, Jan. 2010.

[20] S. Urata and J. C. de la Torre, "Arenavirus budding.," *Adv. Virol.*, vol. 2011, p. 180326, Jan. 2011.

[21] S. R. Radoshitzky, J. Abraham, C. F. Spiropoulou, J. H. Kuhn, D. Nguyen, W. Li, J. Nagel, P. J. Schmidt, J. H. Nunberg, N. C. Andrews, M. Farzan, and H. Choe, "Transferrin receptor 1 is a cellular receptor for New World haemorrhagic fever arenaviruses.," *Nature*, vol. 446, no. 7131, pp. 92–6, Mar. 2007.

[22] P. Aisen, "Transferrin receptor 1.," *Int. J. Biochem. Cell Biol.*, vol. 36, pp. 2137–2143, 2004.

[23] P. H. Gonzalez, P. M. Cossio, R. Arana, J. I. Maiztegui, and R. P. Laguens, "Lymphatic tissue in Argentine hemorrhagic fever: Pathologic features," *Arch. Pathol. Lab. Med.*, vol. 104, pp. 250–254, 1980.

[24] I. S. Lukashevich, R. Maryankova, a S. Vladyko, N. Nashkevich, S. Koleda, M. Djavani, D. Horejsh, N. N. Voitenok, and M. S. Salvato, "Lassa and Mopeia virus replication in human monocytes/macrophages and in endothelial cells: different effects on IL-8 and TNF-alpha gene expression.," *J. Med. Virol.*, vol. 59, no. 4, pp. 552–560, 1999.

[25] D. E. Dylla, D. E. Michele, K. P. Campbell, and P. B. McCray, "Basolateral entry and release of New and Old World arenaviruses from

human airway epithelia.," *J. Virol.*, vol. 82, no. 12, pp. 6034–8, Jun. 2008.

[26] R. L. Guerrant, D. H. Walker, and P. F. Weller, *Tropical Infectious Diseases - Principles, Pathogens and Practice*, 3rd Editio. Saunders - Elsevier, 2011, p. 1155.

[27] M.-L. Moraz and S. Kunz, "Pathogenesis of arenavirus hemorrhagic fevers.," *Expert Rev. Anti. Infect. Ther.*, vol. 9, no. 1, pp. 49–59, 2011.

[28] M. M. E. de Bracco, M. T. Rimoldi, P. M. Cossio, A. Rabinovich, J. I. Maiztegui, G. Carballal, and R. M. Arana, "Argentine Hemorrhagic Fever. Alterations of the Complement System and Anti-Junin-Virus Humoral Response," *New England Journal of Medicine*, vol. 299. pp. 216–221, 1978.

[29] T. G. Terrell, J. L. Stookey, G. a Eddy, and M. D. Kastello, "Pathology of Bolivian hemorrhagic fever in the rhesus monkey.," *Am. J. Pathol.*, vol. 73, no. 2, pp. 477–94, Nov. 1973.

[30] D. H. Walker and F. A. Murphy, "Pathology and pathogenesis of arenavirus infections.," *Curr. Top. Microbiol. Immunol.*, vol. 133, pp. 89–113, 1987.

[31] A. Grant, A. Seregin, C. Huang, O. Kolokoltsova, A. Brasier, C. Peters, and S. Paessler, "Junín virus pathogenesis and virus replication," *Viruses*, vol. 4, no. 10. pp. 2317–2339, Oct-2012.

[32] R. Tesh, "Fiebre hemorrágica venezolana: ocho años de observación," *Acta científica Venez.*, vol. 49, pp. 46–51, 1998.

[33] K. T. McKee, B. G. Mahlandt, J. I. Maiztegui, G. A. Eddy, and C. J. Peters, "Experimental Argentine hemorrhagic fever in rhesus macaques: viral strain-dependent clinical response.," *J. Infect. Dis.*, vol. 152, no. 1, pp. 218–21, Jul. 1985.

[34] C. J. Peters, "Human infection with arenaviruses in the Americas.," *Curr. Top. Microbiol. Immunol.*, vol. 262, pp. 65–74, 2002.

[35] D. Cummins, F. C. Molinas, G. Lerer, J. I. Maiztegui, R. Faint, and S. J. Machin, "A Plasma Inhibitor of Platelet Aggregation in Patients with Argentine Hemorrhagic Fever," *Am. J. Trop. Med. Hyg.*, vol. 42, no. 5, pp. 470–475, May 1990.

[36] M. R. Wilson and C. J. Peters, "Diseases of the central nervous system caused by lymphocytic choriomeningitis virus and other arenaviruses," in *Neurovirology*, 1st ed., vol. 123, Elsevier B.V., 2014, pp. 671–681.

[37] J. I. Maiztegui, N. J. Fernandez, and A. J. de Damilano, "Efficacy of immune plasma in treatment of Argentine haemorrhagic fever and association between treatment and a late neurological syndrome.," 1979.

[38] M. E. Lozano, D. Enria, J. I. Maiztegui, O. Grau, and V. Romanowski, "Rapid diagnosis of argentine hemorrhagic fever by reverse transcriptase

[39] A. R. Trombley, L. Wachter, J. Garrison, V. A. Buckley-Beason, J. Jahrling, L. E. Hensley, R. J. Schoepp, D. a Norwood, A. Goba, J. N. Fair, and D. A. Kulesh, "Comprehensive panel of real-time TaqMan polymerase chain reaction assays for detection and absolute quantification of filoviruses, arenaviruses, and New World hantaviruses.," *Am. J. Trop. Med. Hyg.*, vol. 82, no. 5, pp. 954–60, May 2010.

[40] S. Vieth, C. Drosten, R. Charrel, H. Feldmann, and S. Günther, "Establishment of conventional and fluorescence resonance energy transfer-based real-time PCR assays for detection of pathogenic New World arenaviruses," *J. Clin. Virol.*, vol. 32, pp. 229–235, 2005.

[41] G. Palacios, P. Quan, O. J. Jabado, S. Conlan, D. L. Hirschberg, Y. Liu, J. Zhai, N. Renwick, J. Hui, H. Hegyi, A. Grolla, J. E. Strong, J. S. Towner, T. W. Geisbert, P. B. Jahrling, C. Büchen-Osmond, H. Ellerbrok, M. P. Sanchez-Seco, Y. Lussier, P. Formenty, M. S. T. Nichol, H. Feldmann, T. Briese, and W. I. Lipkin, *Panmicrobial oligonucleotide array for diagnosis of infectious diseases.* 2007.

[42] M. Nakauchi, S. Fukushi, M. Saijo, T. Mizutani, A. E. Ure, V. Romanowski, I. Kurane, and S. Morikawa, "Characterization of monoclonal antibodies to Junin virus nucleocapsid protein and application to the diagnosis of hemorrhagic fever caused by South American arenaviruses.," *Clin. Vaccine Immunol.*, vol. 16, no. 8, pp. 1132–8, Aug. 2009.

[43] A. M. Machado, G. G. Figueiredo, G. M. Campos, M. E. Lozano, A. R. da S. R. Machado, and L. T. M. Figueiredo, "Standardization of an ELISA test using a recombinant nucleoprotein from the Junin virus as the antigen and serological screening for arenavirus among the population of Nova Xavantina, State of Mato Grosso.," *Rev. Soc. Bras. Med. Trop.*, vol. 43, no. 3, pp. 229–33, 2010.

[44] A. E. Ure, P. D. Ghiringhelli, R. D. Possee, S. Morikawa, and V. Romanowski, "Argentine hemorrhagic fever diagnostic test based on recombinant Junín virus N protein," *J. Med. Virol.*, vol. 80, pp. 2127–2133, 2008.

[45] L. E. Alche and C. E. Coto, "Differentiation of junin virus and antigenic variants isolated in vivo by kinetic neutralization assays," *J. Gen. Virol.*, vol. 69, pp. 2123–2127, 1988.

[46] A. A. Kolokoltsov, E. Wang, T. M. Colpitts, S. C. Weaver, and R. A. Davey, "Pseudotyped viruses permit rapid detection of neutralizing antibodies in human and equine serum against Venezuelan equine encephalitis virus," *Am. J. Trop. Med. Hyg.*, vol. 75, pp. 702–709, 2006.

[47] . A. Gross, D. Gitlin, and C. A. Janeway, "The gamma globulins and their clinical significance. IV. Therapeutic uses of gamma globulins.," *N. Engl. J. Med.*, vol. 260, pp. 170–178 concl, 1959.

[48] D. a Enria, A. M. Briggiler, and Z. Sánchez, "Treatment of Argentine hemorrhagic fever," *Antiviral Res.*, vol. 78, no. 1, pp. 132–139, Apr. 2008.

[49] J. I. Maiztegui, N. J. Fernandez, and A. J. de Damilano, "Efficacy of immune plasma in treatment of Argentine haemorrhagic fever and association between treatment and a late neurological syndrome.," *Lancet*, vol. 2, no. 8154, pp. 1216–7, Dec. 1979.

[50] R. W. Sidwell, J. H. Huffman, G. P. Khare, L. B. Allen, J. T. Witkowski, and R. K. Robins, "Broad-spectrum antiviral activity of Virazole: 1-beta-D-ribofuranosyl-1,2,4-triazole-3-carboxamide.," *Science*, vol. 177, no. 1971, pp. 705–706, 1972.

[51] D. a Enria and J. I. Maiztegui, "Antiviral treatment of argentine hemorrhagic fever," *Antiviral Res.*, vol. 23, no. April 1993, pp. 23–31, 1994.

[52] M. Mendenhall, A. Russell, T. Juelich, E. L. Messina, D. F. Smee, A. N. Freiberg, M. R. Holbrook, Y. Furuta, J.-C. de la Torre, J. H. Nunberg, and B. B. Gowen, "T-705 (favipiravir) inhibition of arenavirus replication in cell culture.," *Antimicrob. Agents Chemother.*, vol. 55, no. 2, pp. 782–7, Feb. 2011.

[53] T. C. Bolken, S. Laquerre, Y. Zhang, T. R. Bailey, D. C. Pevear, S. S. Kickner, L. E. Sperzel, K. F. Jones, T. K. Warren, S. Amanda Lund, D. L. Kirkwood-Watts, D. S. King, A. C. Shurtleff, M. C. Guttieri, Y. Deng, M. Bleam, and D. E. Hruby, "Identification and characterization of potent small molecule inhibitor of hemorrhagic fever New World arenaviruses," *Antiviral Res.*, vol. 69, no. 2, pp. 86–97, Feb. 2006.

[54] A. M. Lee, J. M. Rojek, C. F. Spiropoulou, A. T. Gundersen, W. Jin, A. Shaginian, J. York, J. H. Nunberg, D. L. Boger, M. B. a Oldstone, and S. Kunz, "Unique small molecule entry inhibitors of hemorrhagic fever

[55] E. Ortiz-Riaño, N. Ngo, S. Devito, D. Eggink, J. Munger, M. L. Shaw, J. C. de la Torre, and L. Martínez-Sobrido, "Inhibition of arenavirus by A3, a pyrimidine biosynthesis inhibitor.," *J. Virol.*, 2013.

[56] J. A. Pedras-Vasconcelos, M. Puig, C. Sauder, C. Wolbert, M. Ovanesov, D. Goucher, and D. Verthelyi, "Immunotherapy with CpG oligonucleotides and antibodies to TNF-alpha rescues neonatal mice from lethal arenavirus-induced meningoencephalitis.," *J. Immunol.*, vol. 180, pp. 8231–8240, 2008.

[57] M. M. Soares, S. W. King, and P. E. Thorpe, "Targeting inside-out phosphatidylserine as a therapeutic strategy for viral diseases.," *Nat. Med.*, vol. 14, no. 12, pp. 1357–62, Dec. 2008.

[58] A. B. Sánchez, M. Perez, T. Cornu, and J. C. de la Torre, "RNA interference-mediated virus clearance from cells both acutely and chronically infected with the prototypic arenavirus lymphocytic choriomeningitis virus.," *J. Virol.*, vol. 79, pp. 11071–11081, 2005.

[59] I. S. Lukashevich, "Advanced vaccine candidates for Lassa fever.,"

[60] A. S. Parodi, D. J. Greenway, H. R. Rugiero, M. Frigerio, J. M. De la Barrera, N. Mettler, F. Garzon, M. Boxaca, L. Guerrero, and N. Nota, "[Concerning the epidemic outbreak in Junin].," *Dia Med.*, vol. 30, no. 62, pp. 2300–1, Sep. 1958.

[61] D. A. Enria and J. G. Barrera Oro, "Junin virus vaccines.," *Curr. Top. Microbiol. Immunol.*, vol. 263, pp. 239–61, Jan. 2002.

[62] I. Pirosky, J. Zuccarini, E. A. Molinelli, and A. Di Pietro, "Virosis hemorrágica del noroeste bonaerense. II. Recuperacion del virus causal a partir de acaros (Mesostigmata) capturados (1958) en la zona epidemica," *Orientac. Medica*, vol. 8, p. 156, 1959.

[63] C. J. Peters, P. B. Jahrling, C. T. Liu, R. H. Kenyon, K. T. McKeeJr., and J. G. Barrera Oro, "Experimental Studies of Arenaviral Hemorrhagic Fevers," in *Arenaviruses SE- 2*, vol. 134, M. A. Oldstone, Ed. Springer Berlin Heidelberg, 1987, pp. 5–68.

[64] J. G. Barrera Oro and G. A. Eddy, "Characteristics of candidate live attenuated Junín virus vaccine," in *Fourth International Conference on Comparative Virology*, 1982, pp. 17–22.

[65] J. I. Maiztegui, F. Feinsod, A. M. Briggiler, C. J. Peters, D. A. Enría, H. W. Lupton, A. M. Ambrosio, E. Tiano, M. R. Feuillade, G. Gamboa, O. Conti, D. Vallejos, C. MacDonald, and J. G. Barrera Oro, "Inoculation of Argentine volunteers with a live-attenuated Junín virus vaccine," in *VII International Congress of Virology*, 1987, p. 69.

[66] A. M. Ambrosio, L. M. Riera, M. del C. Saavedra, and M. J. Sottosanti, "Preclinical assay of candid #1 vaccine against Argentine Hemorrhagic Fever made in Argentina," *Medicina (B. Aires).*, vol. 65, no. 4, pp. 329–32, Jan. 2005.

[67] D. A. Enria, A. M. Ambrosio, A. M. Briggiler, M. R. Feuillade, and E. Crivelli, "[Candid#1 vaccine against Argentine hemorrhagic fever produced in Argentina. Immunogenicity and safety].," *Medicina (B. Aires).*, vol. 70, no. 3, pp. 215–22, Jan. 2010.

[68] INEVH, "Informe de la XXVI Reunión Anual del Programa Nacional de Control dela FHA," Rosario, Santa Fe, 2012.

[69] R. A. Arribalzaga, "Una nueva enfermedad epidémica a germen desconocido: hipertermia, nefrotóxica, leucopénica y exantemática," *Dia Med.*, vol. 27, pp. 1204–1210, 1955.

[70] J. N. Mills, B. A. Ellis, J. E. Childs, K. T. McKee, J. I. Maiztegui, C. J. Peters, T. G. Ksiazek, and P. B. Jahrling, "Prevalence of infection with Junin virus in rodent populations in the epidemic area of Argentine hemorrhagic fever," *Am. J. Trop. Med. Hyg.*, vol. 51, pp. 554–562, 1994.

[71] G. De Villafañe and S. M. Bonaventura, "Ecological studies in crop fields of the endemic area of Argentine hemorrhagic fever. Calomys musculinus movements in relation to habitat and abundance," *Mammalia*, vol. 51. 1987.

[72] M. C. Weissenbacher, M. S. Sabattini, M. M. Avila, P. M. Sangiorgio, M. R. de Sensi, M. S. Contigiani, S. C. Levis, and J. I. Maiztegui, "Junin virus activity in two rural populations of the Argentine hemorrhagic fever (AHF) endemic area.," *J. Med. Virol.*, vol. 12, no. 4, pp. 273–80, Jan. 1983.

[73] Ministerio de Salud de la Nación, "Programa Nacional de Control de la FHA," Azul, Buenos Aires, Argentina, Fourth Edition, 2007.

[74] Ministery of Health of Argentina, "Informe para la XXVIII Reunión Anual del Programa de Control de la Fiebre Hemorrágica Argentina," 2014.

[75] R. B. Mackenzie, H. K. Beye, L. Valverde, and H. Garron, "Epidemic hemorrhagic fever in Bolivia.," *Am. J. Trop. Med. Hyg.*, vol. 13, pp. 620–625, 1964.

[76] P. a. Webb, "Properties of Machupo virus.," *Am. J. Trop. Med. Hyg.*, vol. 14, pp. 799–802, 1965.

[77] K. M. Johnson, M. L. Kuns, R. B. Mackenzie, P. A. Webb, and C. E. Yunker, "Isolation of Machupo virus from wild rodent Calomys callosus.," *Am. J. Trop. Med. Hyg.*, vol. 15, pp. 103–106, 1966.

[78] J. W. Dragoo, J. Salazar-Bravo, L. J. Layne, and T. L. Yates, "Relationships within the Calomys callosus species group based on amplified fragment length polymorphisms," *Biochem. Syst. Ecol.*, vol. 31, pp. 703–713, 2003.

[79] R. G. Douglas, N. E. D. H. Wiebenga, and R. B. Couch, "Bolivian Hemorrhagic Fever probably transmitted through personal contact," *Am. J. Epidemiol.,* vol. 82, no. 1, pp. 85–91, Jul. 1965.

[80] C. J. Peters, R. W. Kuehne, R. R. Mercado, R. H. L. E. Bow, R. O. Spertzel, M. America, U. S. A. Medi-, M. America, A. A. Divi-, L. Paz, U. S. P. H. Serv-, and P. Fabrega, "Hemorrhagic fever in cochabamba, Bolivia, 1971," vol. 99, no. 6, pp. 425–433, 1974.

[81] K. M. Johnson, "Epidemiology of Machupo virus infection. 3. Significance of virological observations in man and animals.," *Am. J. Trop. Med. Hyg.*, vol. 14, pp. 816–818, 1965.

[82] M. L. Kuns, "Epidemiology of Machupo virus infection. II. Ecological and control studies of hemorrhagic fever.," *Am. J. Trop. Med. Hyg.*, vol. 14, no. 1, pp. 813–816, 1965.

[83] P. E. Kilgore, C. J. Peters, J. N. Mills, P. E. Rollin, L. Armstrong, a. S. Khan, and T. G. Ksiazek, "Prospects for the control of Bolivian hemorrhagic fever.," *Emerg. Infect. Dis.*, vol. 1, no. 3, pp. 97–100, 1995.

[84] P. V. Aguilar, W. Camargo, J. Vargas, C. Guevara, Y. Roca, V. Felices, V. A. Laguna-Torres, R. Tesh, T. G. Ksiazek, and T. J. Kochel, "Reemergence of Bolivian hemorrhagic fever, 2007-2008," *Emerging Infectious Diseases*, vol. 15, no. 9. pp. 1526–1528, 2009.

[85] S. Delgado, B. R. Erickson, R. Agudo, P. J. Blair, E. Vallejo, C. G. Albariño, J. Vargas, J. a Comer, P. E. Rollin, T. G. Ksiazek, J. G. Olson, and S. T. Nichol, "Chapare virus, a newly discovered arenavirus isolated from a fatal hemorrhagic fever case in Bolivia.," *PLoS Pathog.*, vol. 4, no. 4, p. e1000047, Apr. 2008.

[86] T. Lisieux, M. Coimbra, E. S. Nassar, M. N. Burattini, L. T. de Souza, I. Ferreira, I. M. Rocco, A. P. da Rosa, P. F. Vasconcelos, and F. P. Pinheiro, "New arenavirus isolated in Brazil.," *Lancet*, vol. 343, no. 8894, pp. 391–2, Feb. 1994.

[87] T. L. M. Coimbra, E. S. Nassar, M. N. Burattini, L. T. M. De Souza, I. B. Ferreira, I. M. Rocco, A. P. A. Travassos Da Rosa, P. F. C. Vasconcelos, F. P. Pinheiro, J. W. LeDuc, R. Rico-Hesse, J. P. Gonzalez, P. B. Jahrling, and R. B. Tesh, "New arenavirus isolated in Brazil," *Lancet*, vol. 343, pp. 391–392, 1994.

[88] M. Barry, M. Russi, L. Armstrong, D. Geller, R. Tesh, L. Dembry, J. P. Gonzalez, A. S. Khan, and C. J. Peters, *Brief report: treatment of a laboratory-acquired Sabiá virus infection.*, vol. 333. 1995, pp. 294–296.

[89] J. P. Gonzalez, M. D. Bowen, S. T. Nichol, and R. Rico-Hesse, "Genetic characterization and phylogeny of Sabiá virus, an emergent pathogen in Brazil.," *Virology*, vol. 221, no. 2, pp. 318–24, Jul. 1996.

[90] R. Salas, M. E. Pacheco, B. Ramos, M. E. Taibo, E. Jaimes, C. Vasquez, J. Querales, N. de Manzione, O. Godoy, A. Betancourt, F. Araoz, R. Bruzual, J. Garcia, R. B. Tesh, R. Rico-Hesse, and R. E. Shops, "Venezuelan haemorrhagic fever," *Lancet*, vol. 338, no. 8774, pp. 1033–1036, Oct. 1991.

[91] C. F. Fulhorst, T. G. Ksiazek, C. J. Peters, and R. B. Tesh, "Experimental infection of the cane mouse Zygodontomys brevicauda (family Muridae) with guanarito virus (Arenaviridae), the etiologic agent of Venezuelan hemorrhagic fever.," *J. Infect. Dis.*, vol. 180, pp. 966–969, 1999.

[92] C. F. Fulhorst, M. D. Bowen, R. A. Salas, G. Duno, A. Utrera, T. G. Ksiazek, N. M. C. De Manzione, E. De Miller, C. Vasquez, C. J. Peters, and R. B. Tesh, "Natural rodent host associations of Guanarito and Pirital viruses (family Arenaviridae) in central Venezuela," *Am. J. Trop. Med. Hyg.*, vol. 61, no. 2, pp. 325–330, Aug. 1999.

[93] R. B. Tesh, M. L. Wilson, R. Salas, N. M. C. De Manzione, D. Tovar, T. G. Ksiazek, and C. J. Peters, "Field studies on the epidemiology of Venezuelan hemorrhagic fever: Implication of the cotton rat Sigmodon alstoni as the probable rodent reservoir," *Am. J. Trop. Med. Hyg.*, vol. 49, no. February 1992, pp. 227–235, 1993.

[94] N. de Manzione, R. a Salas, H. Paredes, O. Godoy, L. Rojas, F. Araoz, C. F. Fulhorst, T. G. Ksiazek, J. N. Mills, B. a Ellis, C. J. Peters, and R. B. Tesh, "Venezuelan hemorrhagic fever: clinical and epidemiological studies of 165 cases.," *Clin. Infect. Dis.*, vol. 26, pp. 308–313, 1998.

[95] R. B. Tesh, "Viral hemorrhagic fevers of South America.," *Biomed. Rev. del Inst. Nac. Salud*, vol. 22, pp. 287–295, 2002.

[96] R. N. Charrel, H. Feldmann, C. F. Fulhorst, R. Khelifa, R. de Chesse, and X. de Lamballerie, "Phylogeny of New World arenaviruses based on the complete coding sequences of the small genomic segment identified an evolutionary lineage produced by intrasegmental recombination.," *Biochem. Biophys. Res. Commun.*, vol. 296, no. 5, pp. 1118–24, Sep. 2002.

[97] J. T. Paweska, N. H. Sewlall, T. G. Ksiazek, L. H. Blumberg, M. J. Hale, W. I. Lipkin, J. Weyer, S. T. Nichol, P. E. Rollin, L. K. McMullan, C. D. Paddock, T. Briese, J. Mnyaluza, T.-H. Dinh, V. Mukonka, P. Ching, A. Duse, G. Richards, G. de Jong, C. Cohen, B. Ikalafeng, C. Mugero, C.

Asomugha, M. M. Malotle, D. M. Nteo, E. Misiani, R. Swanepoel, and S. R. Zaki, "Nosocomial outbreak of novel arenavirus infection, southern Africa.," *Emerg. Infect. Dis.*, vol. 15, no. 10, pp. 1598–602, Oct. 2009.

[98] T. Briese, J. T. Paweska, L. K. McMullan, S. K. Hutchison, C. Street, G. Palacios, M. L. Khristova, J. Weyer, R. Swanepoel, M. Egholm, S. T. Nichol, and W. I. Lipkin, "Genetic detection and characterization of Lujo virus, a new hemorrhagic fever-associated arenavirus from southern Africa.," *PLoS Pathog.*, vol. 5, no. 5, p. e1000455, May 2009.

In: Hemorrhagic Fever
Editor: Shirley R. Edwards

ISBN: 978-1-63482-791-1

Chapter V

Japanese Encephalitis: Problem of Asia Only?

V. Bostik[1,*]***, M. Salavec***[2]***, R. Sleha***[1]***,***
E. Slehova[3]***, R. Kukla***[3] ***and P. Prasil***[4]
[1]Faculty of Military Health Sciences, University of Defence, Hradec Kralove, Czech Republic
[2]Department of Dermatovenereology, Charles University Medical School and University Hospital, Hradec Kralove, Czech Republic
[3]Faculty of Chemical-Technology, University of Pardubice, Pardubice, Czech Republic
[4]Department of Infectious Diseases, Charles University, Medical School and Faculty Hospital, Hradec Kralove, Czech Republic

Abstract

Japanese encephalitis (JE) is an infectious disease caused by a virus transmitted by blood-sucking arthropods. JE, together with California encephalitis, Saint Louis encephalitis, Central European encephalitis and Russian spring-summer encephalitis, is serious disease affecting the

* Corresponding author: V. Bostik, Faculty of Military Health Sciences, University of Defence, Trebesska 1575, 500 01 Hradec Kralove, Czech Republic. Tel: (420) 973 253 205; E-mail address: vanda.bostikova@unob.cz (Vanda Bostik).

nervous system. After the introduction of universal vaccination against polio, JE is according to the WHO (World Health Organization), worldwide leading disease leading to paretic neuroinfections. It is a vaccine preventable disease typically found in Asia and Western Pacific.

Keywords: Japanese encephalitis, arboviruses, mosquitoes, neuroinfections, vaccination

Characteristics of *Flaviviridae* Family

Japan encephalitis virus belongs to *Flavivirus* genus, family *Flaviviridae*. The term has been derived from Latin word "flavus" – yellow. Beside *Flavivirus* genus two others are included in *Flaviviridae* family, namely *Pestivirus* and *Hepacivirus* [1].

Many others for humans pathogenic viruses, e. g. yellow fever virus, dengue virus and West Nile virus, are included to *Flaviviridae* family [2].

From medical point of view mentioned viral representatives are regarded as source of never-ending problems. Dengue virus is significant morbidity agent worldwide and yellow fever is despite of vaccine availability responsible for epidemics in Africa, as in Latin and South America. West Nile virus is responsible for encephalitis epidemic and febrile disorders every year following its expansion in North America. JE is the main reason of viral encephalitis in Asia and in west Pacific area.

Flavirus contains more than 70 different agents transmitted by mosquito and tick - a half of agents are associated with human diseases. In 16 agents their vector remain unknown. Family classification is based on antigen differences in particular virus. Neutralizing tests divided in 8 groups with 6 of them containing human pathogens are used for typization [4 - 6].

Molecular Structure of *Flaviviruses*

The JE virus is a positive single stranded RNA virus. Nine to twelve thousand bases are encoded by a single polyprotein which consequently split to 3 structural and 7 non-structural proteins. Viral RNA binded in spherical viral capside formed by protein C creates nucleocapsid encapsulated by lipid double layer originating in endoplasmic reticulum. Polymers of viral protein E are anchored to this double layer in immature virions whose binding sites, necessary for fusion with cells, are covered by protein prM. In the maturation process, prM separation and setting of protein E to antiparallel homodimers takes place. Viral size reaches approximately 50 nm in average. Viruses are relatively nonstable, highly sensitive to UV radiation and gamma rays, to detergents, organic solvents (fenol), formaldehyde, alcohol, proteases and lipases. Such substances reliably disintegrate viral capside and effectively inactivate viruses similarly to temperature 56° C treatment for 30 minutes and more. pH level range between 8,4 to 8,8 is essential for viral life. In lower pH levels rapid degradation of viral particles occurs. The above mentioned sensitivity to enzymes is then reason not to contaminate human organism by oral way [7, 8].

JE Genotype Characteristics and Geographical Distribution

The JE virus shows 77% aminoacids homology with West Nile virus, yellow fever virus, viral encephalitis virus and dengue virus. It is highly probable that from evolutional point of view these viruses had one common ancestor and that RNA genome mutations led to its differentiation [7, 9].

Five genotypes marked GI – GV (2 variants GIa and GIb in GI genotype) were described. Though they are congenereous, they succeed in different climate conditions of different climatic zones. Hypothesis published recently supposes original spreading of JE virus from mild climatic zone of Indonesia/Malaysia about 1500. Currently, JE virus occurs in nearly all Asian countries, from Russian Far East to Pakistan in west part of Asia. Some genotypes occur only in southern, other only in northern areas of Asia. Different distribution is associated with different vector kinds in assigned areas and depending on climate type. Phylogenetic studies indicate that genotype IV is the ancestral one. Molecular genetic studies show shift in genotype pattern, in prevalence of some genotypes respectively in last 25 years. In China, Japan, Korea and Vietnam genotype I has been suppressed and replaced by genotype III. Mutation changes of individual genotypes are exactly, obviously as in other flaviviruses, reason for diversity in course of JE in different patients, within geographical areas or in terms of early or late phase of disease epidemic [10 – 16].

JE Incidence and Preventive Measures

Currently, the WHO reports more than 50 000 new JE cases annually. About 20 to 30% of patients die and in 30 to 50% of survivors neurologic and psychiatric consequences as strokes, brain and extrapyramidal symptoms, flexible deformities of upper extremities, hyperextension of lower extremities, speech and teaching disturbances or behavioral problems are present for years. To obtain control of the diseases, the WHO makes effort with impact to endemic areas to work up vaccine campaign consistently and to include JE virus vaccination into national vaccine programmes. Education and distribution of information on stinging insects prevention, i.e. when to reduce outdoor activities (at dawn, at twilight, when is most active and attacks humans outdoors), recommendation for suitable dresses, the use of mosquito nets and repellents – that all is no less important [17, 51].

Child population is affected primarily in endemic areas. Infections confirmed by laboratory methods are present in Asia, 5 to 50 cases per 100 000 pediatric patients respectively. Such value has ever been regarded as lower than real value by the WHO. Still about 1970 approximately 100 000 diseases were recorded only in China. However, vaccine campaign, new cities construction, migration of population from country to urban centres, changes affecting agriculture, controls of mosquito population – all resulted in significant decreases in reported number of cases in China (roughly by 2/3) [17 – 21].

In 2012, thanks to activity of the WHO, 24 Asian countries focused on JE surveillance programme following long stagnation. In 11 countries even immunization programme operates. Philippines, Bhutan and Papua-New Guinea enrolled this surveillance programme. Still in 2011, nineteen of twenty- four countries reported 10 426 JE cases, 8 247 native to India and 1625 cases to China – 95% of all reported cases in total. For all remaining countries less than 150 cases were reported [19].

In an effort to reduce JE cases, the WHO created network of accredited laboratories, introduced training educational courses of lab diagnostics and distributes regularly confirmatory tests to accredited labs. Such approach resulted in significant improvement of JE surveillance. Among others it indicated JE occurrence in Laos. Incidence in Cambodia is considerably higher than suggested initially similarly to Nepal. Vaccines have currently been distributed in these countries by foundation programmes. Due to new, more accurate surveillance data, endemic JE incidence areas were predicted in India,

Sri Lanka, Thailand and in Vietnam and targeted vaccination campaigns are in progress [13, 15, 16, 21, 22].

A zoonotic JE Virus Cycle

JE virus is transmitted during zoonotic cycle between mosquito and vertebrate host (swine, waders) and amplifies in their organism. JE virus affects humans by infected mosquito bite. Only very tiny amount of blood is ingested by vector. The viral threshold concentration in vertebrate needed for infection development is relatively high - 3 – 5 $\log_{10}$ of infectious units are indicated. That is the reason why infection develops in less than 1% of infected individuals. Hosts with insufficient virus concentration are excluded from a cycle.

With the exception of several published cases of intrauterine transmission, the direct human to human transmission is not known. Based on study of other flaviviruses it is supposed that both blood transfusion and organ transplant could be next possible source of human to human transmission anyhow [23 - 25].

JE Virus Vector Types and Their Biotop Characteristics

Mosquito is a transmitter between swine or waders and humans. Most frequently and specifically it is mosquito *C. tritaeniorhynchus* of *Culex* family. It typically occurs in rice fields of Asia. Rice grows as annual plant usually and could deliver harvest in tropical areas for up to 30 years. Traditional method is typical with field flooding during or following in pricking. Such simple method requires persistent water delivery and ground diking.

Other mosquitoes participating in zoonotic cycle are *C. annulus* in Taiwan and Hongkong, *C. vishnui*, *C. gelidus*, *C. pseudovishnui* and *C. fuscocephala* in India and Nepal, *C. gelidus* in Indonesiai and *C. annulirostris* in Pacific region and Australia. *Aedes*, family, specifically *A. togoi* type transmitting JE virus in Russia should also be mentioned.

All these mosquito types are typical with early-evening to night stinging and sucking activity. They prefer to suck animal blood. Their activity peak has been observed and described during sunset outdoor, in nature with minimal build-up area, predominantly in flooded rice fields, at biotopes of meadows with tall grass stand or in bamboo groove and in small slack water slops. Flood imminent areas present the other risk. Most of mosquito outdoors and in mild climate we find from June to November, they are inactive in winter time [17, 26 – 30].

The JE Virus and Travellers from Non-endemic Areas Risk

No cohort according to age is at risk from "imported infection" view (in contrast to above mentioned child population sensitivity to JE virus). The incidence of JE in Asia travelling individuals from non-endemic area is 1 case/1 million travellers. However, in case of travellers long-term persistence in endemic area, risk of infection is the same as for natives. In addition, clinical course of diseases used to be more severe due to low natural immunity. In case of symptom presentation of any neurologic infection as encephalitis, meningitis or acute flaccid paresis in such individual, it is important to inform physician about foreign residence.

Infection imports by travellers are unambiguously influenced by residence site and duration in given areas, seasons of the year depending on mild, tropical or subtropical region and finally by traveler activity type in endemic area. If some of mentioned factors are evaluated as risk factor, prophylactic vaccination must be provided. Vaccination is also important for workers with a risk of infection associated with their professional integration – lab and health system workers, researchers.

In 1973 to 2008 years, 55 JE cases associated with a travel history were published in scientific and in professional journals. Imported cases originated in following countries: Thailand – 19 cases, Indonesia – 8 cases, China – 7 cases, Philippines – 5 cases, Japan – 4 cases and Vietnam – 3 cases. The age indicated in 46 of 55 cases was in 1-91 range, in five cases children under 10 years of age and 10 affected individuals were over 60 years of age. In terms of analyzed group there were 29 men and 22 women, in 4 cases no sex indication was present. All affected individuals were not vaccinated against JE. Ten of presented cases were fatal, 24 survived with health consequences, 12 fully recovered and no result was dated in 9 cases. The most of affected people travelled in the country, lived at farms or travelled on foot in wild open nature [31 – 35].

Clinical Presentation and Diagnostics

Most of JE induced human infections is asymptomatic. Less than 1% infected individuals develops clinical symptoms. Most frequently acute encephalitis occurs. In adults, aseptic meningitis or undefined febrile disorders are recorded.

Incubation period ranges between 5 and 15 days. Clinical presentation begins with fever, cephalea and vomitus. Altered mental condition occurs as well as focal neurologic deficiency, weakness and motility problems – all during several days. Further seizures develop mainly in children, Classical description of JE includes Parkinson syndrome with typical rigid face, tremor, choreoathetoid movements, acute paralysis with symptoms similar to poliomyelitis. Epilepsy, brain hypoxia, intracranial hypertension, brain hernia or aspiration pneumonia are further registered. Such severe complications could result in death of patient.

Japanese encephalitis is a contraindication for pregnancy. Cases of spontaneous abortion and intrauterine infections were detected in association with JE virus. Specific data are from India, presenting 4 abortion cases during first or second trimester in a group of 9 by JEV affected pregnant women. JE virus was successfully isolated in one of four aborted foetus.

Laboratory examination mostly presents non-specific results as mild increase in WBC, mild anemia, hyponatremia, thrombocytopenia and increase in liver enzymes. Lymphocyte pleocytosis with mild hyperproteinemia in cerebrospinal fluid is described.

Brain MRI (Magnetic resonance imaging) shows abnormalities of thalamaus, basal ganglia, mesencephalon, and in spinal cord. Thalamic lesions are mostly described. It is possible to regard such lesions as JE specific, on the other hand they are not regarded as very sensitive sign.

Diagnosis is based on JE specific antibodies evaluation in cerebrospinal fluid (CSF) and detection of viral RNA by PCR method. However, low antibody titers or undetectable viremia and time dependence on clinical specimen sampling could occur, so that these data should not be considered as (critical or crucial?) to exclude JE infection in case of negative results.

Specimen obtained in acute phase delivers positive IgM specific antibodies to JE (capture - MAC ELISA). These antibodies are detectable in CSF in most patients 4 days following clinical symptoms appearance and persist for 7 days. It is always necessary to correlate clinical and laboratory data as well as epidemiologic survey results each other [36 – 40].

Management of JE

Therapy approach is primarily supportive with efforts to prevent complications. There is no casual treatment and quality of supportive care is critical for result. Patients care is focused mainly on stroke prevention, on reducing of brain oedema, fever value decline, secondary infections prevention aimed at death risk and consequent complications reduction.

Due to specific drug absence, non specific antiviral drugs are indicated. Unfortunately, no efficacy of corticosteroids, interferon alpha 2a and ribavirin were demonstrated in clinical trials. The very impracticability of specific antiviral treatment results in high mortality rate and it is extremely necessary to conduct vaccination with other hygienic measures focused on mosquito prevention and disposal [41 – 44, 51].

JE Vaccination

Registered vaccine IXIARO (Novartis, UK) has been available in the EU. It contains inactivated SA 14-14.2 viral strain multiplied in VERO cells tissue culture. Antigen is bind to hydrated aluminium hydroxide.

Vaccine is indicated for JE active immunization adults, in adolescents, in children and in infants more than 2 months of age. Vaccine is administrated *i.m.* into deltoid muscle, in infants to thigh anterolaterally. Two doses of vaccine are delivered in basic scheme (primary immunization), first dose at day 0 and second one at day 28. Each dose contains 0.5 mL of solution, in children up to 3 years of age only 0.25 mL. To achieve protective titers of antibodies it is essential to administer 2 vaccine doses. Most vaccinated individuals according to basic scheme reach protective titer levels to day 35 (7 days after second dose application). Primary immunization should be terminated 1 week before potential exposition at the latest. In individuals with administered first dose of IXARIO vaccine termination of 2-dose vaccine cycle with second dose is fully recommended.

Second dose administered till 11 months after first dose results in high seroconversion level.

The IXIARIO vaccine should never be administered *i.v.* Exceptionally it could be also administered subcutaneously to patients with thrombocytopenia or with bleeding disorders because bleeding could occur in association with *i.m.* administration. Subcutaneous application can result in poor vaccination response and there are no data on clinical efficacy supporting such type of vaccine administration.

Booster vaccine dose in adult is recommended during the second year (i.e. 12-24 months) after primary immunization before a new, potential JE virus exposition. Individuals exposed to permanent risk of Japanese encephalitis (lab personnel or persons residing in endemic areas) should obtain booster dose 12 months following primary immunization.

The IXIARO vaccine is immunogenic sufficiently and following primary immunization protective antibody titers are achieved in all age groups (individuals from 2 months of age, safety and efficacy of IXIARO vaccine in infants under 2 months of age has not been determined yet [45 – 57].

Conclusion

The principal factor for spreading of JE is vector transmitting virus between infected animal and human – a mosquito. In this association it is interesting to realize that more than 3500 different mosquito types are living on our planet (together in 41 families).

For example, mosquitos are responsible for East horse encephalitis virus spreading in Florida. *Aedes triseriatus* spreads La Crosse virus in California, in Persian Gulf countries; *Culex* family then spreads Saint Louis encephalitis virus in North and South America and West Nile virus. Different mosquito types are responsible for West horse encephalitis infection in the USA. *Aedes aegypti* is causative agent for dengue in tropical regions worldwide. This mosquito family has an impact on spreading of Rift Valley fever and of yellow fever. *A. vexans* and *A. caspius* transmit Tahyna virus inducing valtic fever.

It is an unequivocal fact that JE occurrence has gradually been spreading from geographical point of view. Still in the first half of the last century infection occurred in mild climate areas – in Japan, in Korea, in Taiwan and in China. In these areas infection traditionally occurs as seasonal in local epidemics. During last several decades we see it also in Southeast Asia, particularly in India, Bangladesh, Sri Lanka, Papua New Guinea and in Nepal. In areas of subtropical and tropical climatic zone, infection occurs all the year round with a peak during raining season.

The first reports about JE virus occurrence in Australia dated in 90s of 20th century – in wild boars at Mitchell river in Queensland area, in one human individual at the same time. Antibodies directed against JE virus and infected mosquitos of *C. sitiens type* have continuously been detected in wild boars since 2004.

JE virus occurrence spread is obviously result of multifactor action of population mobility, changes in climatic conditions, of ecological factors, agricultural management and domestic animals breeding changes and in modification of birds migration behavior.

References

[1] Ferron F, Bussette C, Dutartre H, Canard B:The modeled structure of the RNA dependent RNA polymerase of GBV-C virus suggests a role for motif E in Flaviviridae RNA polymerases. *BMC Bioinformatics.* 2005; 14(6):255.

[2] Wu YC, Huang YS, Chien LJ, Lin TL, Yueh YY, Tseng WL, Chang KJ, Wang GR. The epidemiology of Japanese encephalitis on Taiwan during 1966-1997. *Am J Trop Med Hyg.* 1999; 61(1):78-84.

[3] www.cdc.gov

[4] Rosen L. The natural history of Japanese encephalitis virus. *Annu Rev Microbiol.* 1986; 40:395 – 414.

[5] Pealer N, Marfin AA, Petersen LR, Lanciotti RS, Page PL, Stramer SL, Stobierski MG, Signs K, Newman B, Kapoor H, Goodman JL, Chamberland ME. Transmission of West Nile virus through blood transfusion in the United States in 2002. *N Engl J Med Hyg.* 2003; 349:1236-45.

[6] Solomon T, Ni H, Beasley DWC, Ekkelenkamp M, Cardosa MJ, Barrett ADT. Origin and evoluion of Japanese encephalitis virus in southeast *Asia. J Virol.* 2003; 77:3091-98.

[7] Elshuber S, Allison SL, Heinz FX, Mandl CW. Cleavage of protein prM is necessary for infection of BHK-21 cells by tick-borne encephalitisvirus. *J Gen Virol.* 2004; 84:183–191.

[8] Luca VC, AbiMansour J, Nelson CA, Fremont DH. Crystal structure of the Japanese Encephalitis virus envelope protein. *J Virol.* 2012; 86(4):2337-2346.

[9] Ferguson M, Johnes S, Li L, Heath A, Barrett A. Effect of genomic variation in the challenge virus on the neutralization titers of recipients of inactivated E vaccines – report of a collaborative study o PRNT50

assays for Japanese encephalitis virus antibodies. *Biologicals.* 2008; 36(2):111-6.

[10] Raengsakulrach B, Nisalak A, Gettaycamin M, Thirawuth V, Young GD, Myint KS, Ferguson LM, Hoke GH, Innis BH, Vaughn DW. Safety, immunogenicity, and protective efficacy of NYVAC-JEV and ALVAC-JEV recombinant Japanese encephalitis vaccines in rhesus monkeys. *Am J Trop Med Hyg.* 1999; 60:343-9.

[11] Poneprasert B. Japanese encephalitis in children in northern Thailand. *Southeast Asian J Trop Med Public Health´.* 1989; 20:599-603.

[12] Ha D, Huong V, Loan H, Thong D, Deubel V. Current situation of Japanese encephalitis in the south of Vietnam. *Trop Med.* 1994; 36:202-14.

[13] Chunsuttiwat S, Warachi P. Japanese encephalitis in Thailand. *Southeast Asian J Trop Med Pub Health.* 1995; 26:43-6.

[14] Joshi D. Current status of Japanese encephalitis in Nepal. *Southeast Asian J Trop Med Pub Health.* 1995, 26:34-40.

[15] Tam N, Yen N. Japanese encephalitis in Sri Lanka. *Southeast Asian J Trop Med Pub Health.* 1995; 26:47-50.

[16] Vitarana T. Japanese encephalitis in Sri Lanka. *Southeast Asian J Trop Med Pub Health.* 1995; 26: 41-2.

[17] Okuno T. An epidemiological review of Japanese encephalitis. *World Health Stat Q.* 1978; 31(2):120-33.

[18] Umenai T, Krzysko R, Bektimirov TA, Assaad FA, Japanese encephalitis: current worldwide status. *Bull World Health Organ.* 1985; 63:625-31.

[19] Encephalitis in Taiwan. I. Introduction and epidemiology. *Am J Trop Med Hyg* 1962, 11: 126-30.

[20] Kono R, Kim KH. Comparative epidemiological features of Japanese encephalitis in the Republic of Korea, China (Taiwan) and Japan. *Bull World Health Organ.* 1969; 40:263-77.

[21] Yongxin Y. Japanese encephalitis in China. *Southeast Asian J Trop Med Pub Health.* 1995; 26:17-21.

[22] Yamada T, Rojanasuphot S, Takagi M, Wungkobkiat S, Hirota T. Studies on an epidemic of Japanese emcephalitis in the northern region of Thailand in 1969 and 1970. *Biken J.* 1971; 14:267-96.

[23] Bernard P, Jambaud E, Berbineau A, Brunot J, Flechaire A. Japanese encephalitis an ecptional imported arbovirus. *Presse Med.* 1998; 27:1327.

[24] Simpson DIH, Smith CEG, Marshall TF, et al. Arbovirus infecions in Sarawak: the role of the domestic pig. *Trans R Soc Trop Med Hyg* 1976,70:66-72.

[25] CDC. Japanese encephalitis vaccines: recommendations of the Advisory Committee on Immunization Practices (ACIP). *MMRW,* 2010; 59:1-27.

[26] Igarashi A. Epidemiology and control of Japanese encephalitis. *World Health Stat Q.* 1992; 45:299-305.

[27] Keiser J, Maltese MF, Erlanger TE, Bos R, Tanner M, Singer BH, Utzinger J. Effect of irrigated rice agriculture on Japanese encephalitis, including challenges and opportunities for integrated vector management. *Acta Trop.* 2005; 95:40-57.

[28] Olson JG, Ksiazek TG, Tan R, Atmosoedjono S, Lee VH, Converse JD Correlation o opulation indices of female *Culex tritaeniorhynchus* with Japanese encephalitis viral activity in Kapuk, Indonesia. *Southeast Asian J Trop Med Pub Health.* 1985; 16:337-42.

[29] Reisen WK, Aslamkhan M, Basio RG. The effects of climatic patterns and agricultural pracices on the population dynamics of *Culex tritaeniorhynchus* in Asia. *Southeast Asian J Trop Med Pub Health.* 1976; 61-71.

[30] Grossman RA, Edelman R, Gould DJ. Study of Japanese encephalitis virus in Chiangmia Valley, Thailand. *Am J Epidemiol.* 1974; 100:69-76.

[31] Gingrich JB, Nisalak A, Latendresse JR, Sattabongkot JH, Hoke CH, Pomsdhit J, Chantalakana C, Satayaphanta C, Uechiewcharnkit K, Innis BL. Japanese encephalitis virus in Bankok: actors influencing vector infections in three suburban communities. *J Med Entomol.* 1992; 29:436-44.

[32] Kari K., Liu W., Gautama K., Mammen MP, Clemens JD, Nisalak A, Subrata K, Kim HK, Xu, ZY. A hospital-based surveillance for Japanese encephalitis in Bali, Indonesia. *BMC Med.* 2006; 4:8.

[33] Bista MB, Shrestha JM. Epidemiological situation of Japanese encephalitis in Nepal. *Jnma.* 2005; 44:51-6.

[34] Hanna JN, Ritchie S, Phillips DA, Lee JM, Hills SL, van den Hurk AF, Pyke AT, Johansen CA, Mackenzie JS. Japanese encephalitis in north Queensland, Australia, 1998. *Med J Austr.* 1999; 170:533-6.

[35] Hanna JN, Ritchie S, Phillips DA, Shield J, Mackenzie JS, Poidinger M, McCall BJ, Mill PJ. An outbreak of Japanese encephalitis in the Torres Strait, Australia 1995. *Med J Austr.*1996; 165:256-60.

[36] SolomonT, Vaughn DW Pathogenesis and clinical features of Japanese encephalitis and West Nile infection. *Curr Top Microbiol Immunol.* 2002; 267:171-94.

[37] Wat G, Jongsakul K. Acute undifferentiated fever caused by infection with Japanese encephalitis virus. *Am J Trop Med Hyg.* 2003; 68: 704-6.

[38] Kuwayama M, Ito M, Takao S, Shimazu Y, Fukuda S, Miyazaki K, Kurane I, Takasaki T. Japanese encephalitis virus in meningitis patients, *Japan. Emer Infect Dis.* 2005; 11:471-3.

[39] Halstead SB, Grosz CR. Subclinical Japanese encephalitis. Infection of Americans with limited residence in Korea. *Am J Hyg.* 1962; 75:190-201.

[40] Benenson MW, Top FH, Gresso W, Ames C, Altstatt LB. The virulence to man of Japanese eephalitis virus in Thailand. *Am J Trop Med Hyg.* 1975; 24:974-80.

[41] Potula R, Badrinath S, Srinivasan S. Japanese encephalitis in and around Pondicherry, South India – a clinical appraisal and prognostic indicators for the outcome. *J Trop Pediatr.* 2003; 49:48-53.

[42] Gajanana A, Thenmozhi V, Samuel PP, Reuben R. A community based study of subclinical flavivirus infection in children in an area of Tamil Nadu, India, where Japanese encephalitis is endemic. *Bull World Health Organ.* 1995; 73:237-44.

[43] Libraty DH, Nisalak A, Endy TP, Suntayakorn S, Vauhn DW, Innis BL. Clinical and immunological risk factors for severe disease in Japanese encephalitis. *Trans R Soc Trop Med Hyg.* 2002; 96:173-8.

[44] Grossman RA, Edelman R, Willhight M, Pantuwatana S, Udomsakdi S. Study of Japanese encephalitis virus in Thailand. *Am J Epidemiol.* 1973; 98:133-49.

[45] Geraghty CM, McCarthy JS. Japanese encephalitis vaccine – is it being sufficiently used in travelers. *Med Aus.* 2004; 181:269-70.

[46] Hanson JP, Taylor CT, Richards R, Smith IL, Boutlis CS. Japanese encephalitis acquired near Port Moresby-implications for residents and travelers to Papua New Guinea. *Med J Aust.* 2004; 181:282-3.

[47] Ferguson M, Kurane I, Wimalaratne O, Shin J, Wood D. WHO informal consultation on the scientific basis of specifications for production and control of inactivated Japanese encephalitis vaccines for human use, Geneva, Switzerland,2006. *Vaccine.* 2007; 25:5233-43.

[48] WHO. Global Advisory Committee on Vaccine Safety, 2005. *Wkly Epidemiol Rec.* 2005; 80:242-7.

[49] Teitelbaum P. Expert opinion on vaccination of travelers against Japanese encephalitis. *J Trav Med.* 2009; 16:441.

[50] Rojanasuphot S, Mai P, Srijaggrawalwon A, Panthumachinda B, Nimmannitya S. Implementation of simultaneous Japanese encephalitis vaccination in the expanded programme on immunization of infants. *Mosquito-Borne Diseases Bulletin.* 1992; 9: 86-92.

[51] http://www.path.org/projects/JE_

[52] Diagana M, Preux PM, Dumas M. Japanese encephalitis revisited. *J Neurol Sci.* 2007 Nov 15;262(1-2):165-70.

[53] Schuller E, Jilma B, Voicu V, et al. Long-term immunogenicity of the new Vero cell-derived, inactivated Japanese encephalitis virus vaccine IC51 Six and 12 month results of a multicenter follow-up phase 3 study. *Vaccine* 2008; 26: 4382-6.

[54] Schuller E, Klade CS, Woelfl G, et al. Comparison of a single, high-dose vaccination regimen to the standard regimen for the investigational Japanese encephalitis vaccine, IC51: A randomized, observer-blind, controlled Phase 3 study. *Vaccine* 2009; 27: 2188-2193.

[55] Kaltenboeck et al. Immunogenicity and safety of IXIARO (IC51) in a Phase II study in healthy Indian children between 1 and 3 years of age. *Vaccine* 2010;28:834-9.

[56] Dubischar-Kastner et al. *Interim Safety and Immunogenicity Data for the Inactivated Japanese Encephalitis Vaccine IXIARO®,* IC51, in Children from JE non-endemic countries. Presented at the 4th Northern European Conference on Travel Medicine, June 2012, Abstract P.9. Abstract available at http://nectm.com/wp-content/uploads/BookofAbstracts.pdf.

[57] Dubischar-Kastner et al. Safety and Immunogenicity of the Inactivated Japanese Encephalitis Vaccine IXIARO®, IC51, in Filipino Children aged 2 months to <18 years. Presented at the 4th Northern European Conference on Travel Medicine, June 2012, Abstract P.9. Abstract available at http://nectm.com/wp-content/uploads/BookofAbstracts.pdf.

Index

E

F

G

H

I

J

K

L

M

N

O

P

T

U

V

W

Y

Z